HIGH TRIGLYCERIDES DIET
Cookbook for Beginners

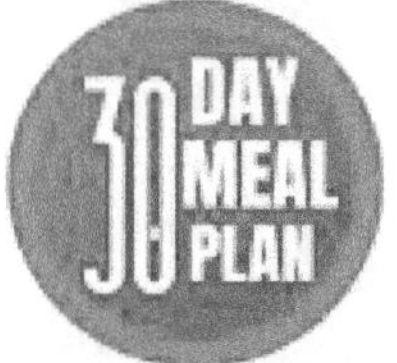

Flavorful Recipes and Expert Tips to Lower Triglycerides, Enhance Heart Health, and Boost Your Wellness

Cheryl C. Smith

<u>GET ACCESS TO MORE OF MY BOOKS BY SCANNING THE QR CODE BELOW</u>

TABLE OF CONTENTS

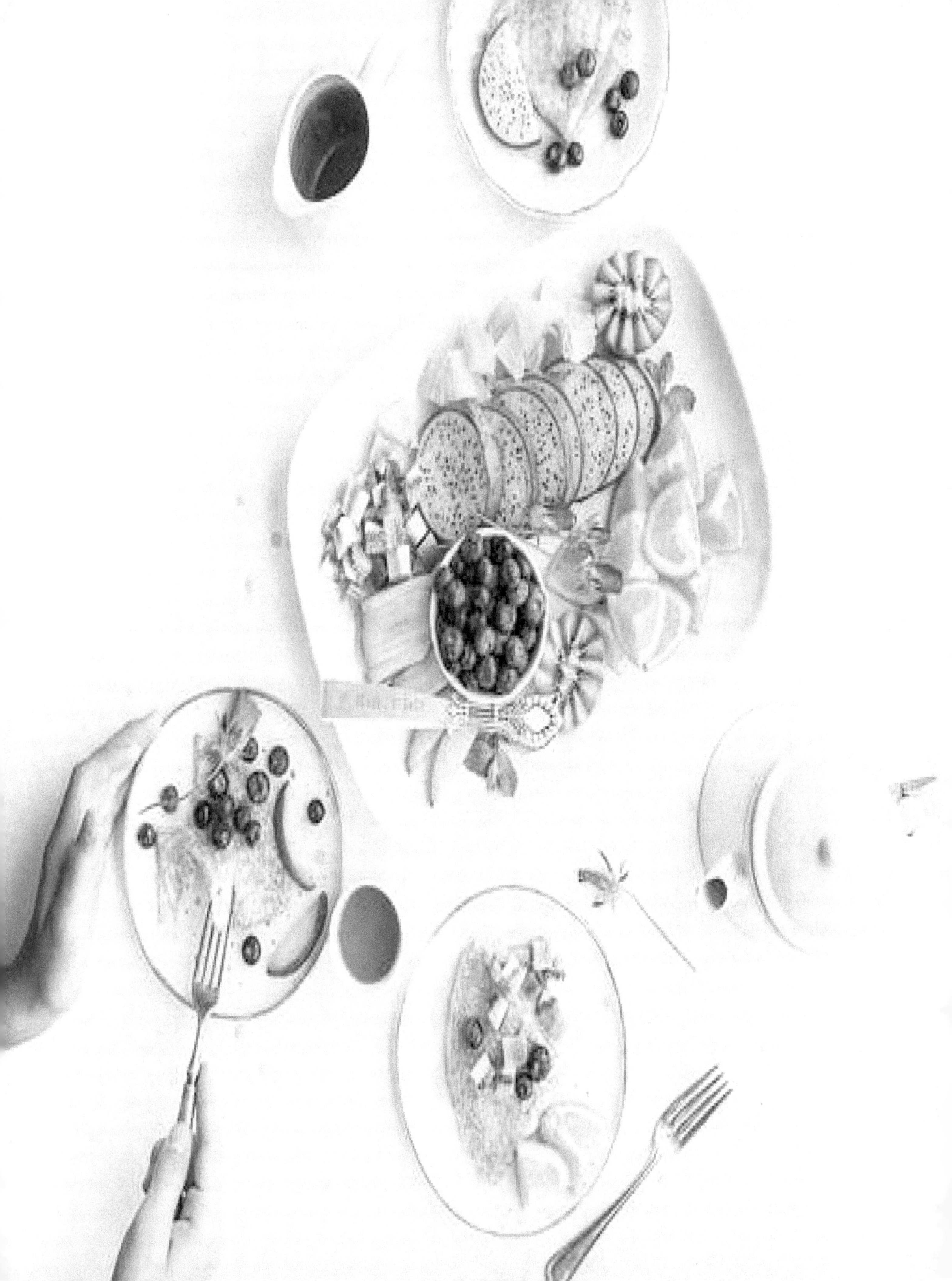

Having high triglyceride levels is a condition that can contribute to heart disease. There is no specific diet for losing weight if you have high triglycerides. Rather, you need to follow a healthy eating plan that meets your nutritional needs while helping you lower your triglycerides. This High Triglyceride Diet Cookbook provides crucial information and support to help you manage y our condition. Gain the tools you need to take control and create a diet that works for you.

CHAPTER 1: UNDERSTANDING HIGH TRIGLYCERIDES

Firstly, it is important to understand that triglycerides are not 'bad." They are a fuel that your body uses to make energy. However, triglycerides are involved in metabolic syndrome. If you consume too many calories, more fat circulates in the blood, causing an upward spiral of fatty acid buildup, which then leads to high triglycerides. High triglycerides also pose a risk for heart disease, as individuals with elevated blood fats (a condition in which triglycerides and cholesterol are elevated in the blood) often have high levels of fats in their arteries.

You are at risk for high triglyceride levels if you are over 40, consume a lot of fat, or have diabetes. In addition, obesity, excessive alcohol intake, and kidney or liver disease can cause high triglyceride levels. Some medications may also raise the triglyceride levels in your blood.

What Are High Triglycerides?

Triglycerides are a type of fat found in the blood, which the body uses for energy. A person's triglyceride levels can be too high or too low. These levels measure the amount of triglycerides in the blood. High levels mean that the body may not be using all the calories eaten in a day. More calories are turned into triglycerides, leading to high amounts in the blood. This can cause disease. For instance, high levels may cause a person to be more likely to get heart disease. This is the most common cause of high levels. Uncontrolled diabetes can also cause high levels. Other causes can include kidney disease, drinking too much alcohol, hypothyroidism, liver disease, and some medicines.

Causes and Symptoms

Symptoms:

Although no symptoms are strictly associated with high levels of triglycerides, very high levels can cause pancreatitis (severe abdominal pain, nausea, and vomiting) or xanthomas (yellowish deposits of fat under the skin, particularly around the eyes).

<u>**Causes:**</u>

There can be a lot of causes for high levels of triglyceride. The causes of high triglyceride levels are numerous and include both reversible and irreversible factors. Some causes include type 2 diabetes, hypothyroidism (underactive thyroid), kidney disease, liver disease, proteinuria (abnormal loss of protein in the urine), multiple myeloma, obesity, pregnancy, family history, high alcohol consumption, and estrogen therapy. Many serious diseases are related to high levels of triglyceride, so the people with High levels of triglyceride should pay more attention to their body.

Diagnostic Procedures

There are several different diagnostic procedures your physician may employ to investigate excessive triglyceride levels. One of the most common procedures is a blood test. A blood sample is drawn from your arm and tested to determine the levels of cholesterol and triglycerides in your blood. This test is known as lipoprotein analysis. It is often performed after at least a 12-hour fast and provides two important numbers: total cholesterol and LDL-C levels. Also known as the "bad" cholesterol because high levels can lead to heart disease. It's measured in milligrams (mg) of cholesterol per deciliter of blood (dL). HDL-C levels are also a key part of your cholesterol count, though they are not usually included in the LDL measurements of the traditional cholesterol test. HDL-C is known as the "good" cholesterol because high levels can reduce the risk of cardiovascular diseases.

There are also tests that determine your HDL-C level. These tests also measure the levels of good cholesterol (HDL-C) in your blood. The tests are best done after true fasting since glucose in the blood puts off the collection time of the proteins of interest. Ideally, a 'normal' HDL level is 50 or higher for women, and 40 or higher for men. A lower HDL level increases the risk for heart disease. Age also plays a role in cholesterol health, as both levels elevate as women are young, and men as they grow older.

The Dangers of High Triglycerides

Excessive triglycerides raise the risk of the following conditions by hardening the arteries or thickening the arterial walls (atherosclerosis):

- **Heart Disease:** High blood pressure, elevated cholesterol, and high triglycerides are common risk factors for cardiovascular disease.
- **Stroke:** Blood clot development and atherosclerosis can cause strokes.
- **Pancreatitis:** Acute inflammation of the pancreas may result from abnormally elevated triglyceride levels.
- **Metabolic Syndrome:** This cluster of disorders raises the risk of diabetes, heart disease, and stroke. It also includes high blood pressure, excessive blood sugar, excess body fat around the waist, and abnormal cholesterol levels.

CHAPTER 2: STRATEGIES TO LOWER TRIGLYCERIDES

When you have high triglycerides, eating to lower them is important. Did you know you can do this simply by choosing different foods? While high cholesterol checks measure LDL and HDL, a blood test for high triglycerides measures a type of fat that affects the body similarly. High triglycerides can raise the risk of heart disease; a lower LDL count reflects the amount of bad cholesterol, while a higher HDL count is beneficial for good heart health. Fortunately, even a small reduction in foods that spike blood sugar can significantly reduce fat and lower your triglyceride levels.

Lifestyle Changes and Healthy Habits

Lifestyle changes: To maintain healthy levels of triglycerides, monitor the intake of high-caloric, high-sugar (simple carbohydrates), and starchy foods, as well as alcohol and weight gain. Additionally, engaging in mild to moderate exercise or physical activity, such as a 30-minute walk most days of the week, along with a fiber-enriched diet, helps reduce triglyceride levels and provides protection against heart disease and other chronic conditions such as type 2 diabetes, obesity, and hypertension.

Healthy habits: Eating regular, balanced meals that include lean protein, whole grains, a variety of fruits and vegetables, healthy fats such as seeds and nuts (monounsaturated and omega-3 fatty acids), skinless poultry, and fish helps maintain normal triglyceride levels. Additionally, practice active stress relief techniques such as deep breathing, meditation, and engaging in regular hobbies to maintain normal blood pressure.

Diet: Ultimately, consuming fewer calories, especially those packed with protein and high-fiber foods, along with regular exercise, are key elements for maintaining healthy triglyceride levels. This is where the High Triglyceride Diet Cookbook for Beginners can help by offering mouthwatering recipes suited for the beginner cook and emphasizing healthy eating habits.

Importance of Physical Activity

Engaging in moderate to vigorous physical activity is an important part of any weight-loss program. The number of calories burned during exercise will obviously exceed the number of calories burned by just sitting around doing nothing. Generally, the more vigorous the exercise, the more calories you will burn. Whether or not this activity is part of a well-matched diet, the structure of the activity and the integration of the diet can help obese individuals achieve a negative energy balance.

<u>**Types of Exercise:**</u>

- **Aerobic Activities:**
  - Participate in moderate-intensity aerobic activity for at least 150 minutes each week. Examples of such exercises include walking, jogging, swimming, and cycling.
- **Strength Training:**
  - Incorporate strength training exercises at least twice a week to build muscle and boost your metabolism.

- **Flexibility and Balance:**
  - Activities such as yoga and tai chi improve overall physical health and complement both aerobic and strength exercises.

Detecting High Triglycerides Early

High triglycerides, medically known as hypertriglyceridemia, are a condition that requires medical attention. It is often diagnosed through a blood test known as a lipid panel. The lipid profile provides a comparison of cholesterol levels and triglyceride levels, which are types of fat, also known as lipids, in your blood. This detection is important because high triglycerides can increase the risk of atherosclerosis, which is the thickening and hardening of your arteries that can lead to blockages, heart attack, stroke, or heart disease. Sometimes, this condition may not show any physical symptoms, and you may be unaware of it.

It is generally measured as follows:

Normal — Less than 150 mg/dL

Borderline-High — Between 150 - 199 mg/dL

High — Between 200 - 499 mg/dL

Very high — Over 500 mg/dL

When detected early, high triglycerides can be easily managed with simple dietary and lifestyle modifications. These include regular exercise, avoiding sugary processed foods, eating unsaturated fats, and consuming omega-3 fatty acids.

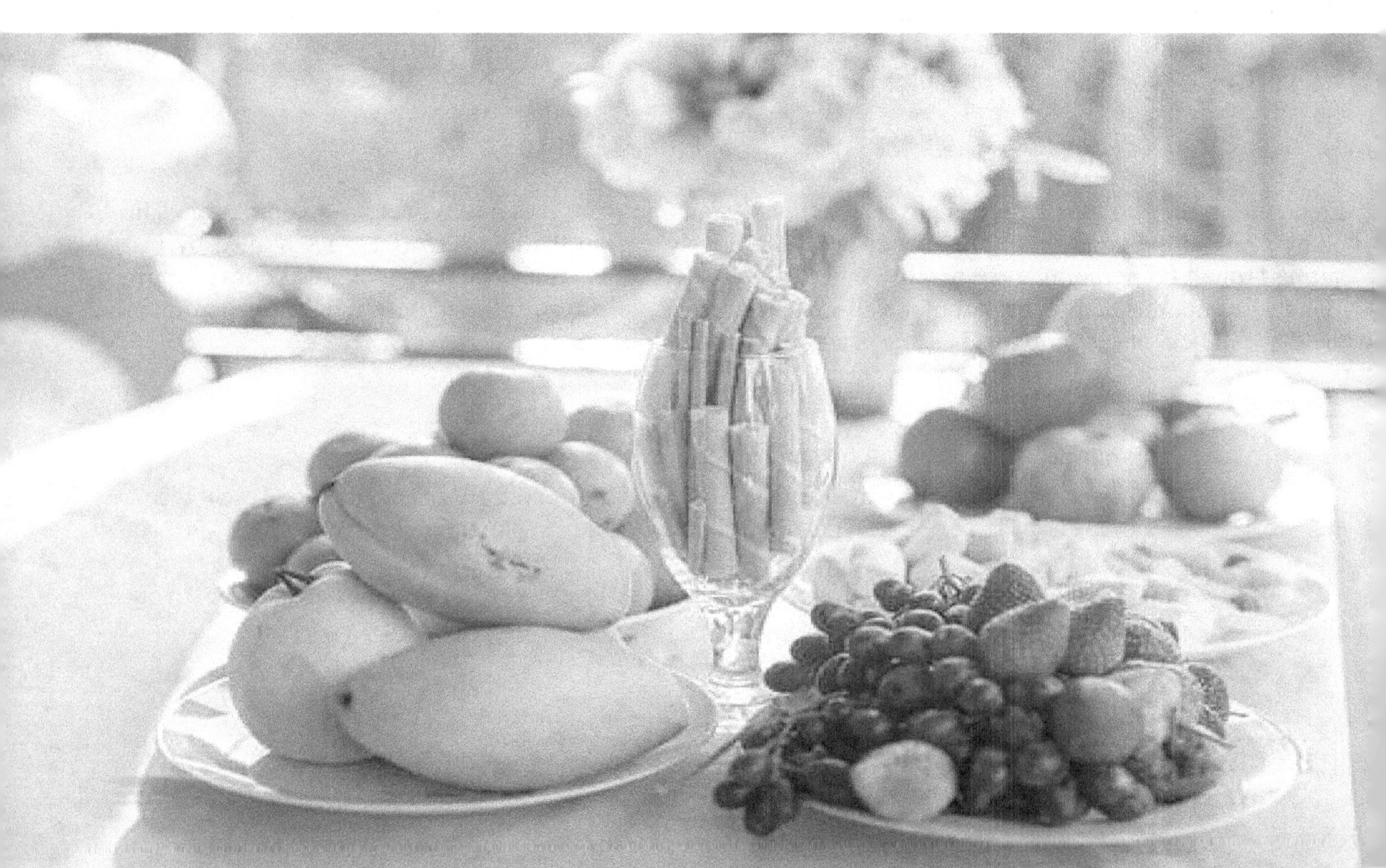

The latest nutrition guidelines clearly illustrate the relationship between what we eat and disease prevention, management, and overall health. Poor nutrition is a risk factor for many chronic diseases, including cancer, heart disease, diabetes, and stroke.

Foods to Include

Incorporating the right foods into your diet can help manage and lower triglyceride levels effectively. Consider the following nutrient-dense options:

Healthy Fats

1. **Omega-3 Fatty Acids:** Found in fatty fish like salmon, mackerel, sardines, and trout. Also available in flaxseeds, chia seeds, and walnuts.
2. **Monounsaturated Fats:** Sources include olive oil, avocados, almonds, and peanuts.
3. **Polyunsaturated Fats:** Found in sunflower oil, soybean oil, and fish oil supplements.

High-Fiber Foods

1. **Fruits:** Berries, apples, pears, oranges, and bananas.
2. **Vegetables:** Leafy greens, broccoli, carrots, and Brussels sprouts.
3. **Whole Grains:** Oatmeal, quinoa, brown rice, and whole wheat bread.
4. **Legumes:** Beans, lentils, and chickpeas.

Lean Proteins

1. **Poultry:** Skinless chicken and turkey.
2. **Fish:** Fatty fish rich in omega-3 fatty acids.
3. **Plant-Based Proteins:** Tofu, tempeh, and legumes.

Dairy

1. **Low-Fat or Non-Fat Options:** Skim milk, low-fat yogurt, and reduced-fat cheese.

Nuts and Seeds

- **Healthy Options:** Almonds, walnuts, chia seeds, and flaxseeds.

Foods to Avoid

Here's the list of foods that increase the levels of triglycerides. These foods are best avoided in a diet when diagnosed with high triglycerides.

Sugary Foods and Beverages

1. **Sugary Drinks:** Soda, fruit juices, and energy drinks.
2. **Sweets:** Candy, cakes, cookies, and pastries.
3. **Processed Sugars:** Table sugar, high-fructose corn syrup, and other added sugars.

<u>**Refined Carbohydrates**</u>

1. **White Bread and Pasta:** Made from refined flour.
2. **White Rice:** Choose brown or wild rice instead.
3. **Processed Snacks:** Chips, crackers, and other packaged snacks.

<u>**Unhealthy Fats**</u>

1. **Trans Fats:** Found in many fried foods, baked goods, and processed snacks.
2. **Saturated Fats:** Limit red meat, full-fat dairy products, and certain oils like coconut oil and palm oil.
3. **Fried Foods:** Avoid deep-fried foods and opt for baked or grilled options.

<u>**Alcohol**</u>

- **Limit Intake:** Excessive alcohol consumption can significantly raise triglyceride levels.

Balanced Diet Tips

Following these tips can help you maintain a balanced diet that supports healthy triglyceride levels:

<u>**Portion Control**</u>

1. **Watch Serving Sizes:** Use smaller plates and be mindful of portion sizes to avoid overeating.
2. **Frequent, Small Meals:** Eating smaller, more frequent meals can help maintain steady blood sugar levels.

<u>**Meal Planning**</u>

1. **Plan Ahead:** Create weekly meal plans to ensure balanced and nutritious meals.
2. **Grocery Lists:** Make a list before shopping to avoid impulse buys of unhealthy foods.

<u>**Cooking Methods**</u>

1. **Healthy Cooking Techniques:** Opt for grilling, baking, steaming, or sautéing instead of frying.
2. **Use Healthy Oils:** Cook with olive oil or other healthy fats instead of butter or lard.

<u>**Hydration**</u>

1. **Drink Plenty of Water:** Staying hydrated helps your body function optimally and can help control appetite.

<u>**Reading Labels**</u>

- **Check Nutritional Information:** Read food labels to avoid hidden sugars and unhealthy fats.
- **Ingredient Lists:** Opt for foods with minimal and recognizable ingredients.

How Diet Affects Triglycerides

Triglycerides are a type of fat in the bloodstream. Although they transport fatty acids, which are important for energy, high levels can lead to atherosclerosis. In addition to genetic factors, this condition can also be promoted by dietary habits, alcohol abuse, smoking, obesity, hypertension, diabetes, and a lack of exercise. The excess of these fats is deposited mainly in visceral fat, increasing the risk of heart and blood vessel disease.

Essential Nutrients for Lowering Triglycerides

To effectively lower triglyceride levels, focus on incorporating the following essential nutrients into your diet:

- **Omega-3 Fatty Acids:** Found in fatty fish like salmon, mackerel, and sardines, as well as in flaxseeds and walnuts, omega-3s can significantly reduce triglycerides.
- **Fiber:** High-fiber foods such as oats, legumes, fruits, and vegetables help reduce the absorption of fat and sugar in the bloodstream.
- **Healthy Fats:** Unsaturated fats, like those found in avocados, olive oil, and nuts, can help improve lipid profiles.
- **Antioxidants:** Berries, leafy greens, and other colorful fruits and vegetables are rich in antioxidants, which can reduce inflammation and improve heart health.
- **Lean Proteins:** Opt for sources like chicken, turkey, tofu, and legumes to provide essential nutrients without the added saturated fats found in red meats.

Meal Planning Tips for Beginners

Meal planning is one of the essential strategies to help reduce your blood triglycerides and to maintain a healthy diet overall. However, preparing and planning your meals can come with many challenges. Here are some meal planning tips for beginners to help make preparing and planning your meals as stress-free as possible.

1. **Plan Ahead:** Set up time every week to organize your snacks and meals. This will assist you in choosing better options and warding off unhealthy last-minute decisions.
2. **Balance Your Plate:** Aim for a balanced plate with a mix of lean protein, healthy fats, and fiber-rich carbohydrates.
3. **Portion Control:** Be mindful of portion sizes to avoid overeating, which can lead to elevated triglyceride levels.
4. **Stay Hydrated:** Drink water in large quantities throughout the day. Limit alcohol intake and avoid sugar-filled beverages.
5. **Batch Cooking:** Prepare larger quantities of healthy meals and store them for quick and easy access during the week.
6. **Healthy Swaps:** Make simple swaps, such as using whole grains instead of refined grains and opting for healthier cooking methods like grilling or baking instead of frying.
7. **Read Labels:** Be aware of hidden sugars and unhealthy fats in packaged foods by reading nutrition labels carefully.

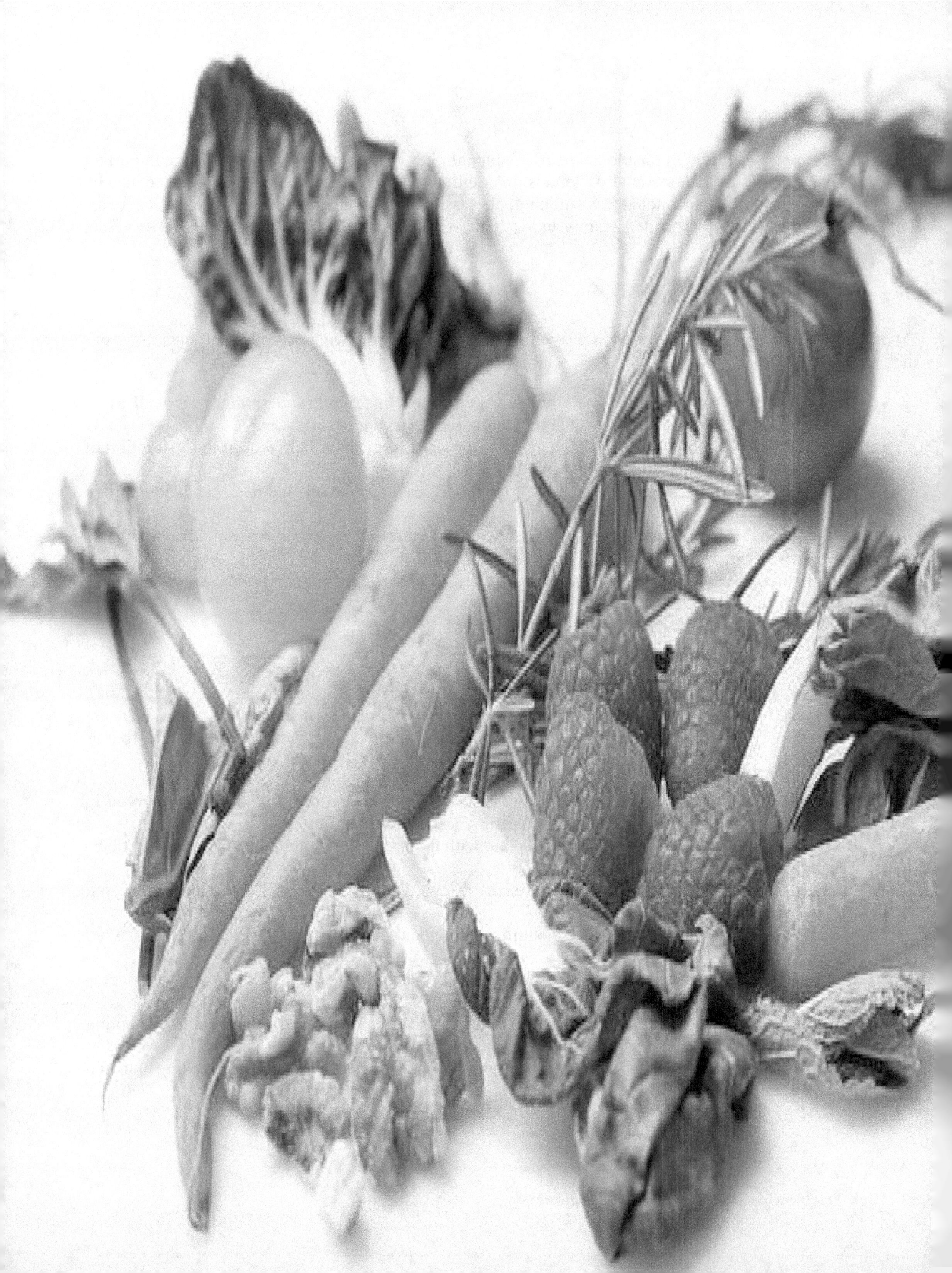

BREAKFAST RECIPES

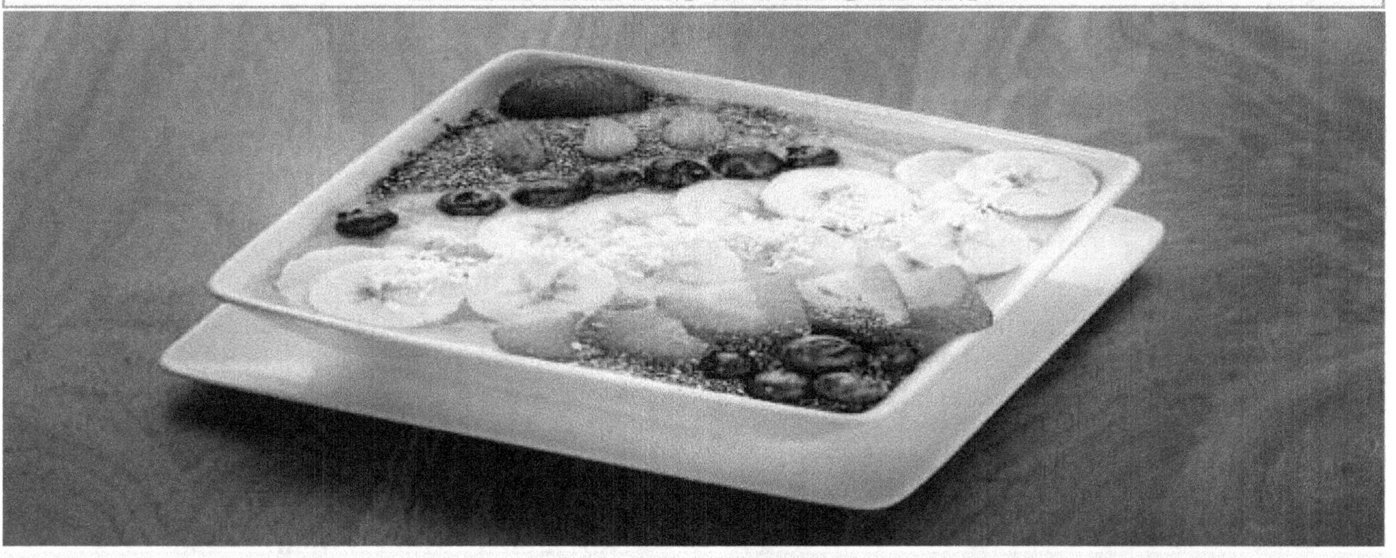

Avocado and Spinach Smoothie

Prep Time: 5 minutes | **Cooking Time:** 0 minutes | **Servings:** 2

Ingredients:

- 1 ripe avocado
- 1 cup fresh spinach
- 1 banana
- 1 cup unsweetened almond milk
- 1 tablespoon chia seeds
- 1 teaspoon honey (optional)
- 1/2 cup ice cubes

Instructions:

1. Cut the avocado in half, remove the pit, and scoop the flesh into a blender.
2. Add the fresh spinach, banana, almond milk, chia seeds, and honey (if using) to the blender.
3. Add ice cubes to the blender.
4. Blend on high until smooth and creamy.
5. Pour into glasses and serve immediately.

Nutritional Information: Calories: 250 | Protein: 4g | Carbs: 30g | Fat: 14g | Fiber: 10g

Greek Yogurt with Berries and Chia Seeds

Prep Time: 5 minutes | **Cooking Time:** 0 minutes | **Servings:** 1

Ingredients:

- 1 cup Greek yogurt
- 1/2 cup mixed berries (strawberries, blueberries, raspberries)
- 1 tablespoon chia seeds
- 1 teaspoon honey (optional)
- 1 tablespoon sliced almonds

Instructions:

1. Place the Greek yogurt in a bowl.
2. Top with mixed berries.
3. Sprinkle chia seeds and sliced almonds on top.
4. Drizzle with honey if desired.
5. Serve immediately.

Nutritional Information: Calories: 200 | Protein: 15g | Carbs: 25g | Fat: 7g | Fiber: 5g

Oatmeal with Flaxseed and Almonds

⏱ **Prep Time:** 5 minutes | 🔍 **Cooking Time:** 5 minutes | 🍽 **Servings:** 1

🛒 **Ingredients:**

- 1/2 cup rolled oats
- 1 cup water or unsweetened almond milk
- 1 tablespoon ground flaxseed
- 1 tablespoon sliced almonds
- 1/2 teaspoon cinnamon
- 1 teaspoon honey (optional)
- 1/4 cup fresh berries (optional)

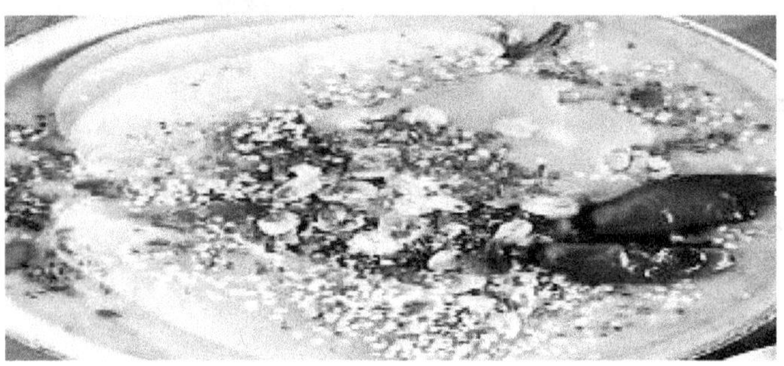

📋 **Instructions:**

1. In a small pot, bring water or almond milk to a boil.
2. Add rolled oats and reduce heat to a simmer. Cook for 5 minutes, stirring occasionally.
3. Stir in ground flaxseed and cinnamon.
4. Pour the oatmeal into a bowl.
5. Top with sliced almonds, honey, and fresh berries if desired.
6. Serve immediately.

🍱 **Nutritional Information:** Calories: 220 | Protein: 7g | Carbs: 35g | Fat: 7g | Fiber: 8g

Scrambled Egg Whites with Vegetables

⏱ **Prep Time:** 5 minutes | 🔍 **Cooking Time:** 5 minutes | 🍽 **Servings:** 1

🛒 **Ingredients:**

- 4 egg whites
- 1/4 cup diced bell peppers
- 1/4 cup diced tomatoes
- 1/4 cup spinach leaves, chopped
- Salt and pepper to taste
- 1 teaspoon olive oil

📋 **Instructions:**

1. Heat olive oil in a non-stick skillet over medium heat.
2. Add diced bell peppers and cook for 2 minutes.
3. Add diced tomatoes and chopped spinach, cooking for an additional 2 minutes.
4. In a bowl, whisk the egg whites with salt and pepper.
5. Pour the egg whites into the skillet with the vegetables.
6. Stir continuously until the egg whites are fully cooked.
7. Serve immediately.

🍱 **Nutritional Information:** Calories: 120 | Protein: 20g | Carbs: 5g | Fat: 3g | Fiber: 2g

Quinoa Breakfast Bowl

⏱ **Prep Time:** 10 minutes | 🔍 **Cooking Time:** 15 minutes | 🍽 **Servings:** 2

🛒 **Ingredients:**

- 1/2 cup quinoa
- 1 cup water
- 1/4 cup almond milk
- 1 tablespoon honey

- 1/2 teaspoon vanilla extract
- 1/2 cup mixed berries
- 1 tablespoon chia seeds
- 1 tablespoon sliced almonds

Instructions:

1. Rinse quinoa under cold water.
2. In a pot, bring water to a boil and add quinoa. Reduce heat, cover, and simmer for 15 minutes or until quinoa is tender and water is absorbed.
3. Stir in almond milk, honey, and vanilla extract.
4. Divide the quinoa into bowls.
5. Top with mixed berries, chia seeds, and sliced almonds.
6. Serve immediately.

Nutritional Information: Calories: 250 | Protein: 8g | Carbs: 45g | Fat: 6g | Fiber: 7g

Whole Wheat Toast with Avocado Spread

Prep Time: 5 minutes | **Cooking Time:** 2 minutes | **Servings:** 1

Ingredients:

- 1 slice whole wheat bread
- 1/2 ripe avocado
- 1 teaspoon lemon juice
- Salt and pepper to taste
- 1/4 teaspoon red pepper flakes (optional)

Instructions:

1. Toast the whole wheat bread to your desired level of crispiness.
2. In a small bowl, mash the avocado with lemon juice, salt, and pepper.
3. Spread the mashed avocado mixture onto the toasted bread.
4. Sprinkle red pepper flakes on top if desired.
5. Serve immediately.

Nutritional Information: Calories: 180 | Protein: 4g | Carbs: 20g | Fat: 10g | Fiber: 6g

Berry and Nut Parfait

Prep Time: 5 minutes | **Cooking Time:** 0 minutes | **Servings:** 1

Ingredients:

- 1 cup Greek yogurt
- 1/2 cup mixed berries (strawberries, blueberries, raspberries)
- 1 tablespoon honey
- 2 tablespoons granola
- 1 tablespoon chopped nuts (almonds, walnuts, or pecans)

Instructions:

1. In a glass or bowl, layer half of the Greek yogurt.
2. Add half of the mixed berries on top of the yogurt.
3. Drizzle with half of the honey.
4. Add the remaining Greek yogurt, followed by the rest of the berries.
5. Drizzle with the remaining honey.
6. Top with granola and chopped nuts.
7. Serve immediately.

Nutritional Information: Calories: 250 | Protein: 14g | Carbs: 35g | Fat: 8g | Fiber: 5g

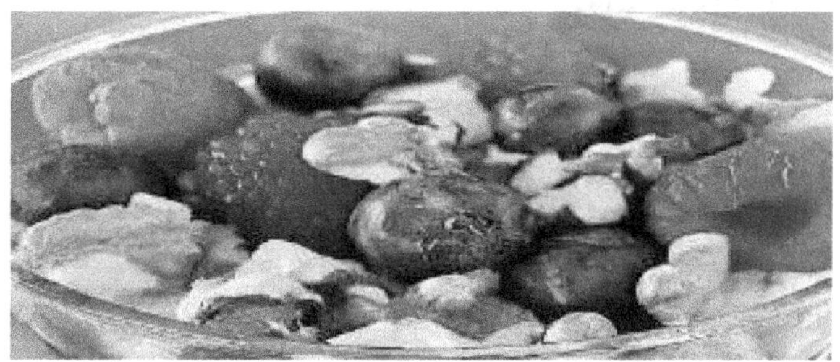

Veggie-Packed Frittata

⏱ **Prep Time:** 10 minutes | 🔍 **Cooking Time:** 20 minutes | 🍽 **Servings:** 4

🛒 **Ingredients:**

- 6 large eggs
- 1/4 cup milk
- 1 cup diced bell peppers
- 1/2 cup diced onions
- 1/2 cup chopped spinach
- 1/4 cup shredded low-fat cheese
- Salt and pepper to taste
- 1 tablespoon olive oil

📋 **Instructions:**

1. Preheat the oven to 375°F (190°C).
2. In a large bowl, whisk together the eggs and milk. Season with salt and pepper.
3. Heat olive oil in an oven-safe skillet over medium heat.
4. Add the bell peppers and onions, cooking until soft, about 5 minutes.
5. Stir in the chopped spinach and cook until wilted, about 2 minutes.
6. Pour the egg mixture over the vegetables and sprinkle with shredded cheese.
7. Transfer the skillet to the preheated oven and bake for 15 minutes, or until the eggs are set.
8. Remove from the oven and let cool slightly before slicing.
9. Serve warm.

🍚 **Nutritional Information:** Calories: 180 | Protein: 12g | Carbs: 6g | Fat: 12g | Fiber: 2g

Green Detox Smoothie

⏱ **Prep Time:** 5 minutes | 🔍 **Cooking Time:** 0 minutes | 🍽 **Servings:** 2

🛒 **Ingredients:**

- 1 cup kale leaves, chopped
- 1 cup spinach
- 1 green apple, cored and chopped
- 1/2 cucumber, chopped
- 1/2 lemon, juiced
- 1 tablespoon chia seeds
- 1 cup water
- 1/2 cup ice cubes

📋 **Instructions:**

1. Add kale, spinach, green apple, cucumber, lemon juice, chia seeds, water, and ice cubes to a blender.
2. Blend on high until smooth and creamy.
3. Pour into glasses and serve immediately.

🍚 **Nutritional Information:** Calories: 130 | Protein: 3g | Carbs: 29g | Fat: 2g | Fiber: 8g

Chia Seed Pudding with Fresh Fruit

⏱ **Prep Time:** 5 minutes | 🔍 **Cooking Time:** 0 minutes | 🍽 **Servings:** 2

📋 **Instructions:**

1. In a bowl, whisk together chia seeds, almond milk, honey, and vanilla extract.
2. Cover and refrigerate for at least 4 hours or overnight.
3. Stir the pudding and divide into bowls.
4. Top with mixed fresh fruit.
5. Serve immediately.

🛒 **Ingredients:**

- 1/4 cup chia seeds
- 1 cup unsweetened almond milk
- 1 tablespoon honey
- 1/2 teaspoon vanilla extract
- 1/2 cup mixed fresh fruit (berries, kiwi, mango)

🍚 **Nutritional Information:** Calories: 180 | Protein: 4g | Carbs: 30g | Fat: 7g | Fiber: 10g

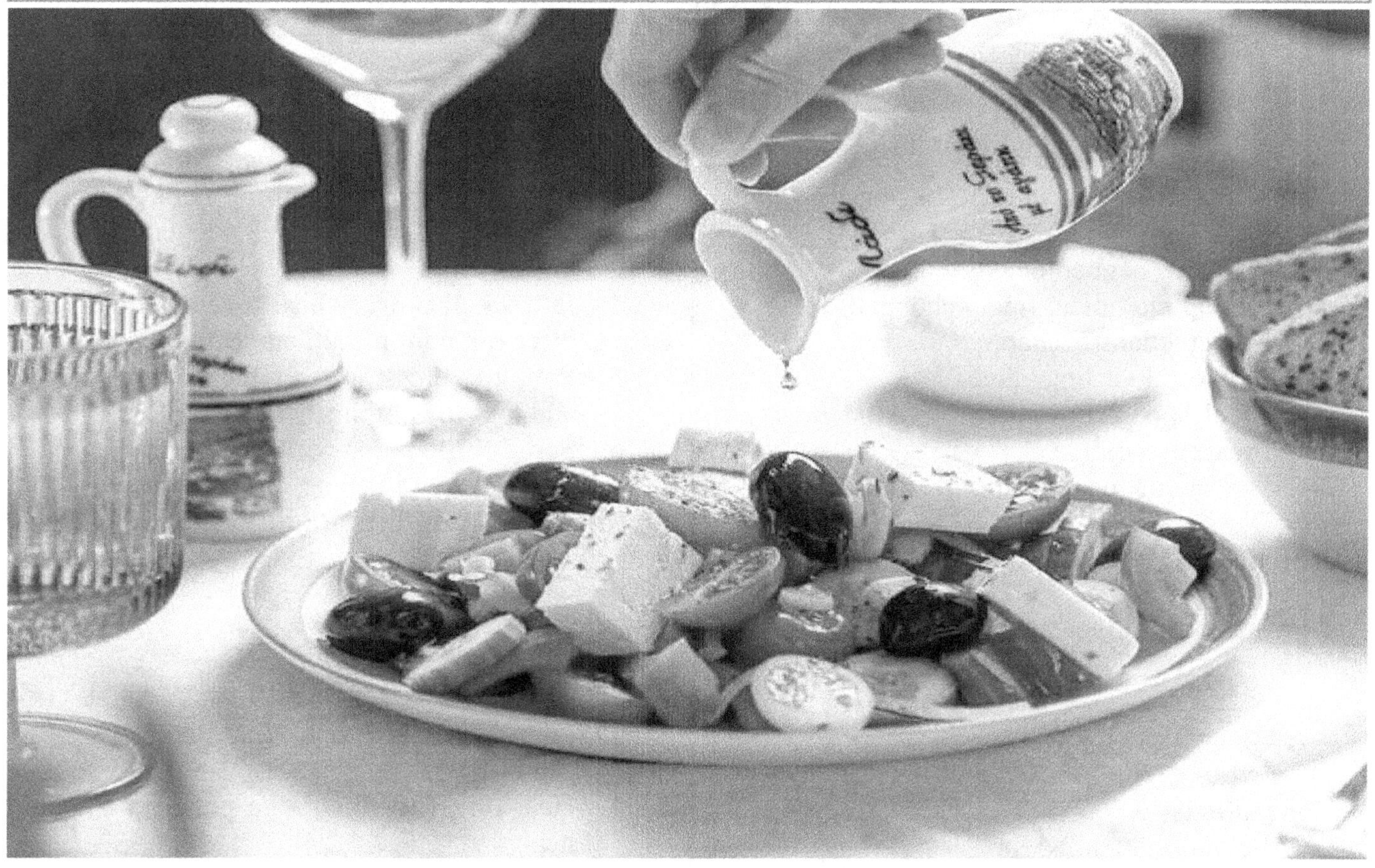

Grilled Chicken Salad with Olive Oil Dressing

Prep Time: 15 minutes | **Cooking Time:** 10 minutes | Servings: 2

Ingredients:

- 2 boneless, skinless chicken breasts
- 4 cups mixed greens (lettuce, spinach, arugula)
- 1/2 cup cherry tomatoes, halved
- 1/4 cup red onion, thinly sliced
- 1/4 cup cucumber, sliced
- 1/4 cup feta cheese, crumbled
- 2 tablespoons olive oil
- 1 tablespoon balsamic vinegar
- Salt and pepper to taste

Instructions:

1. Season the chicken breasts with salt and pepper.
2. Heat a grill or grill pan over medium-high heat. Grill the chicken breasts for about 5 minutes on each side, or until fully cooked.
3. Let the chicken rest for a few minutes, then slice into strips.
4. In a large bowl, combine mixed greens, cherry tomatoes, red onion, cucumber, and feta cheese.
5. In a small bowl, whisk together olive oil and balsamic vinegar. Season with salt and pepper.
6. Drizzle the dressing over the salad and toss to combine.
7. Top the salad with grilled chicken slices and serve immediately.

Nutritional Information: Calories: 350 | Protein: 35g | Carbs: 12g | Fat: 20g | Fiber: 4g

Quinoa and Black Bean Salad

⏱ Prep Time: 10 minutes | **🔍 Cooking Time:** 15 minutes | **🍽 Servings:** 4

🛒 Ingredients:

- 1 cup quinoa
- 1 can (15 oz) black beans, rinsed and drained
- 1 cup corn kernels (fresh or frozen)
- 1 red bell pepper, diced
- 1/4 cup red onion, finely chopped
- 1/4 cup cilantro, chopped
- 3 tablespoons lime juice
- 2 tablespoons olive oil
- 1 teaspoon cumin
- Salt and pepper to taste

📋 Instructions:

1. Rinse the quinoa under cold water.
2. In a pot, bring 2 cups of water to a boil. Add the quinoa, reduce heat, cover, and simmer for 15 minutes or until water is absorbed.
3. In a large bowl, combine cooked quinoa, black beans, corn, red bell pepper, red onion, and cilantro.
4. In a small bowl, whisk together lime juice, olive oil, cumin, salt, and pepper.
5. Pour the dressing over the quinoa mixture and toss to combine.
6. Serve chilled or at room temperature.

🍱 Nutritional Information: Calories: 280 | Protein: 9g | Carbs: 45g | Fat: 8g | Fiber: 8g

Lentil Soup with Kale

⏱ Prep Time: 10 minutes | **🔍 Cooking Time:** 30 minutes | **🍽 Servings:** 4

🛒 Ingredients:

- 1 cup dried lentils, rinsed
- 6 cups vegetable broth
- 1 onion, diced
- 2 carrots, diced
- 2 celery stalks, diced
- 3 garlic cloves, minced
- 2 cups chopped kale
- 1 can (14.5 oz) diced tomatoes
- 1 teaspoon dried thyme
- 1 teaspoon cumin
- 1 tablespoon olive oil
- Salt and pepper to taste

📋 Instructions:

1. Heat olive oil in a large pot over medium heat.
2. Add onion, carrots, and celery, and cook until vegetables are tender, about 5 minutes.
3. Stir in garlic, thyme, and cumin, cooking for another minute.
4. Add lentils, vegetable broth, and diced tomatoes. Bring to a boil, then reduce heat and simmer for 25 minutes.
5. Stir in kale and cook for an additional 5 minutes.
6. Season with salt and pepper to taste.
7. Serve hot.

🍱 Nutritional Information: Calories: 200 | Protein: 11g | Carbs: 35g | Fat: 4g | Fiber: 12g

Turkey and Avocado Wrap

⏱ Prep Time: 10 minutes | **🔍 Cooking Time:** 0 minutes | **🍽 Servings:** 1

🛒 Ingredients:

- 1 whole wheat tortilla
- 3 slices deli turkey breast
- 1/2 avocado, sliced
- 1/4 cup spinach leaves
- 1/4 cup shredded carrots
- 1 tablespoon hummus
- Salt and pepper to taste

Instructions:

1. Lay the whole wheat tortilla flat on a clean surface.
2. Spread the hummus evenly over the tortilla.
3. Layer the turkey slices, avocado, spinach, and shredded carrots on top.
4. Season with salt and pepper to taste.
5. Roll the tortilla tightly into a wrap.
6. Slice in half and serve immediately.

Nutritional Information: Calories: 320 | Protein: 20g | Carbs: 30g | Fat: 15g | Fiber: 8g

Spinach and Feta Stuffed Peppers

Prep Time: 15 minutes | **Cooking Time:** 25 minutes | **Servings:** 4

Ingredients:

- 4 large bell peppers
- 1 cup cooked quinoa
- 1 cup fresh spinach, chopped
- 1/2 cup feta cheese, crumbled
- 1/4 cup red onion, diced
- 1 teaspoon dried oregano
- 1 tablespoon olive oil
- Salt and pepper to taste

Instructions:

1. Preheat the oven to 375°F (190°C).
2. Cut the tops off the bell peppers and remove the seeds and membranes.
3. In a large bowl, combine cooked quinoa, spinach, feta cheese, red onion, oregano, olive oil, salt, and pepper.
4. Stuff the bell peppers with the quinoa mixture.
5. Place the stuffed peppers in a baking dish and cover with foil.
6. Bake for 20 minutes, then remove the foil and bake for an additional 5 minutes.
7. Serve warm.

Nutritional Information: Calories: 200 | Protein: 8g | Carbs: 25g | Fat: 8g | Fiber: 6g

Baked Salmon with Asparagus

Prep Time: 10 minutes | **Cooking Time:** 20 minutes | **Servings:** 2

Ingredients:

- 2 salmon fillets
- 1 bunch asparagus, trimmed
- 1 lemon, sliced
- 2 tablespoons olive oil
- 1 teaspoon garlic powder
- Salt and pepper to taste

Instructions:

1. Preheat the oven to 400°F (200°C).
2. Place the salmon fillets on a baking sheet lined with parchment paper.
3. Arrange the asparagus around the salmon.
4. Drizzle olive oil over the salmon and asparagus.
5. Sprinkle garlic powder, salt, and pepper over the salmon and asparagus.
6. Top the salmon with lemon slices.
7. Bake for 20 minutes or until the salmon is cooked through and the asparagus is tender.
8. Serve immediately.

Nutritional Information: Calories: 350 | Protein: 30g | Carbs: 8g | Fat: 22g | Fiber: 4g

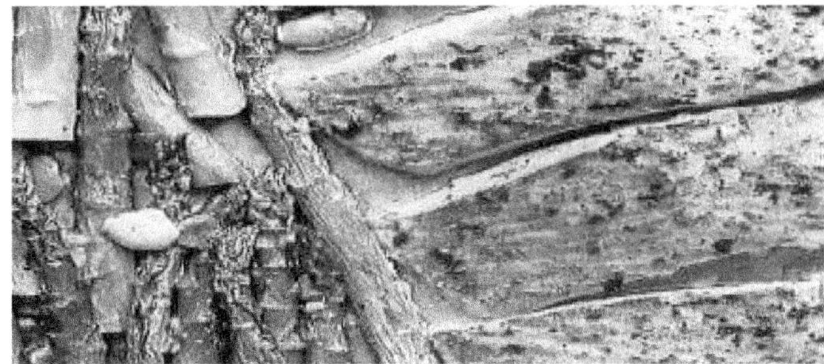

Chickpea and Veggie Stir-Fry

⏱ Prep Time: 10 minutes | **🍳 Cooking Time:** 15 minutes | **🍽 Servings:** 4

🛒 Ingredients:

- 1 can (15 oz) chickpeas, rinsed and drained
- 1 red bell pepper, sliced
- 1 yellow bell pepper, sliced
- 1 zucchini, sliced
- 1 cup broccoli florets
- 2 tablespoons soy sauce (low sodium)
- 1 tablespoon olive oil
- 1 teaspoon ginger, grated
- 2 garlic cloves, minced
- 1 tablespoon sesame seeds
- Salt and pepper to taste

📋 Instructions:

1. Heat olive oil in a large skillet over medium-high heat.
2. Add garlic and ginger, cooking for 1 minute until fragrant.
3. Add bell peppers, zucchini, and broccoli to the skillet. Cook for 5-7 minutes until vegetables are tender-crisp.
4. Stir in chickpeas and soy sauce, cooking for another 5 minutes.
5. Sprinkle with sesame seeds and season with salt and pepper.
6. Serve immediately.

🥗 Nutritional Information: Calories: 250 | Protein: 10g | Carbs: 30g | Fat: 10g | Fiber: 8g

Tuna Salad with Greek Yogurt Dressing

⏱ Prep Time: 10 minutes | **🍳 Cooking Time:** 0 minutes | **🍽 Servings:** 2

🛒 Ingredients:

- 1 can (5 oz) tuna in water, drained
- 1/4 cup Greek yogurt
- 1 tablespoon lemon juice
- 1 celery stalk, diced
- 1/4 cup red onion, diced
- 1 tablespoon fresh dill, chopped
- Salt and pepper to taste
- Mixed greens for serving

📋 Instructions:

1. In a bowl, combine the tuna, Greek yogurt, lemon juice, celery, red onion, and fresh dill.
2. Season with salt and pepper to taste.
3. Serve the tuna salad over a bed of mixed greens.
4. Serve immediately.

🥗 Nutritional Information: Calories: 150 | Protein: 20g | Carbs: 5g | Fat: 5g | Fiber: 1g

Whole Grain Pita with Hummus and Veggies

⏱ Prep Time: 10 minutes | **🍳 Cooking Time:** 0 minutes | **🍽 Servings:** 2

📋 Instructions:

1. Cut the whole grain pitas in half to create pockets.
2. Spread hummus inside each pita half.
3. Stuff each pita with cucumber, cherry tomatoes, shredded carrots, red bell pepper, and mixed greens.
4. Serve immediately.

🛒 Ingredients:

- 2 whole grain pitas
- 1/2 cup hummus
- 1/4 cup cucumber, sliced
- 1/4 cup cherry tomatoes, halved
- 1/4 cup shredded carrots
- 1/4 cup red bell pepper, sliced
- 1/4 cup mixed greens

🥗 Nutritional Information: Calories: 300 | Protein: 10g | Carbs: 45g | Fat: 10g | Fiber: 8g

Mediterranean Farro Salad

⏱ Prep Time: 10 minutes | **🔍 Cooking Time:** 25 minutes | **🍽 Servings:** 4

🛒 Ingredients:

- 1 cup farro
- 2 cups water
- 1/2 cup cherry tomatoes, halved
- 1/2 cup cucumber, diced
- 1/4 cup red onion, diced
- 1/4 cup Kalamata olives, pitted and sliced
- 1/4 cup feta cheese, crumbled
- 2 tablespoons olive oil
- 2 tablespoons lemon juice
- 1 teaspoon dried oregano
- Salt and pepper to taste

📋 Instructions:

1. Rinse farro under cold water.
2. In a pot, bring 2 cups of water to a boil. Add farro, reduce heat, cover, and simmer for 25 minutes or until farro is tender.
3. Drain any excess water and let farro cool.
4. In a large bowl, combine cooked farro, cherry tomatoes, cucumber, red onion, olives, and feta cheese.
5. In a small bowl, whisk together olive oil, lemon juice, oregano, salt, and pepper.
6. Pour the dressing over the farro mixture and toss to combine.
7. Serve chilled or at room temperature.

🥗 **Nutritional Information:** Calories: 320 | Protein: 8g | Carbs: 45g | Fat: 12g | Fiber: 8g

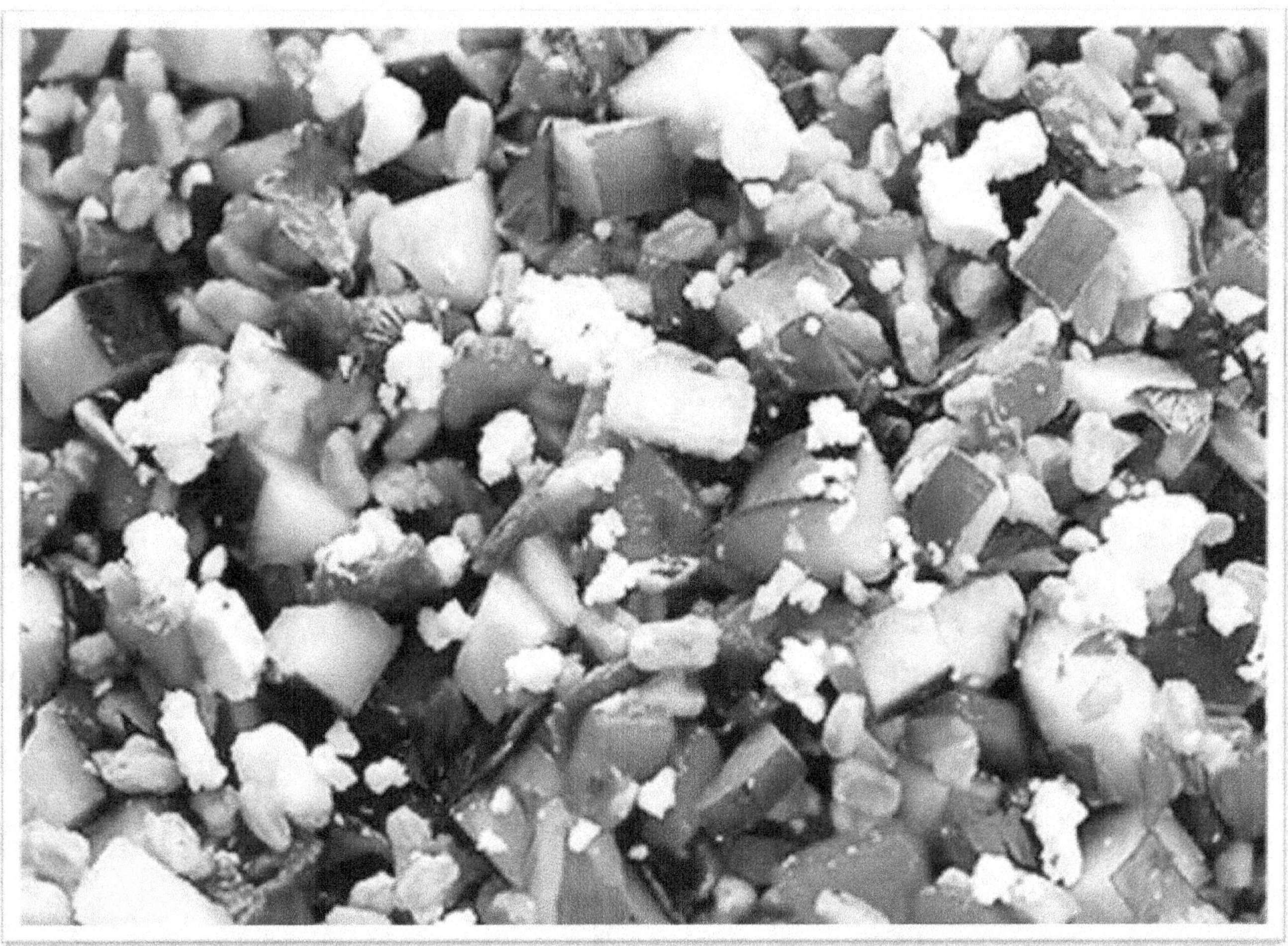

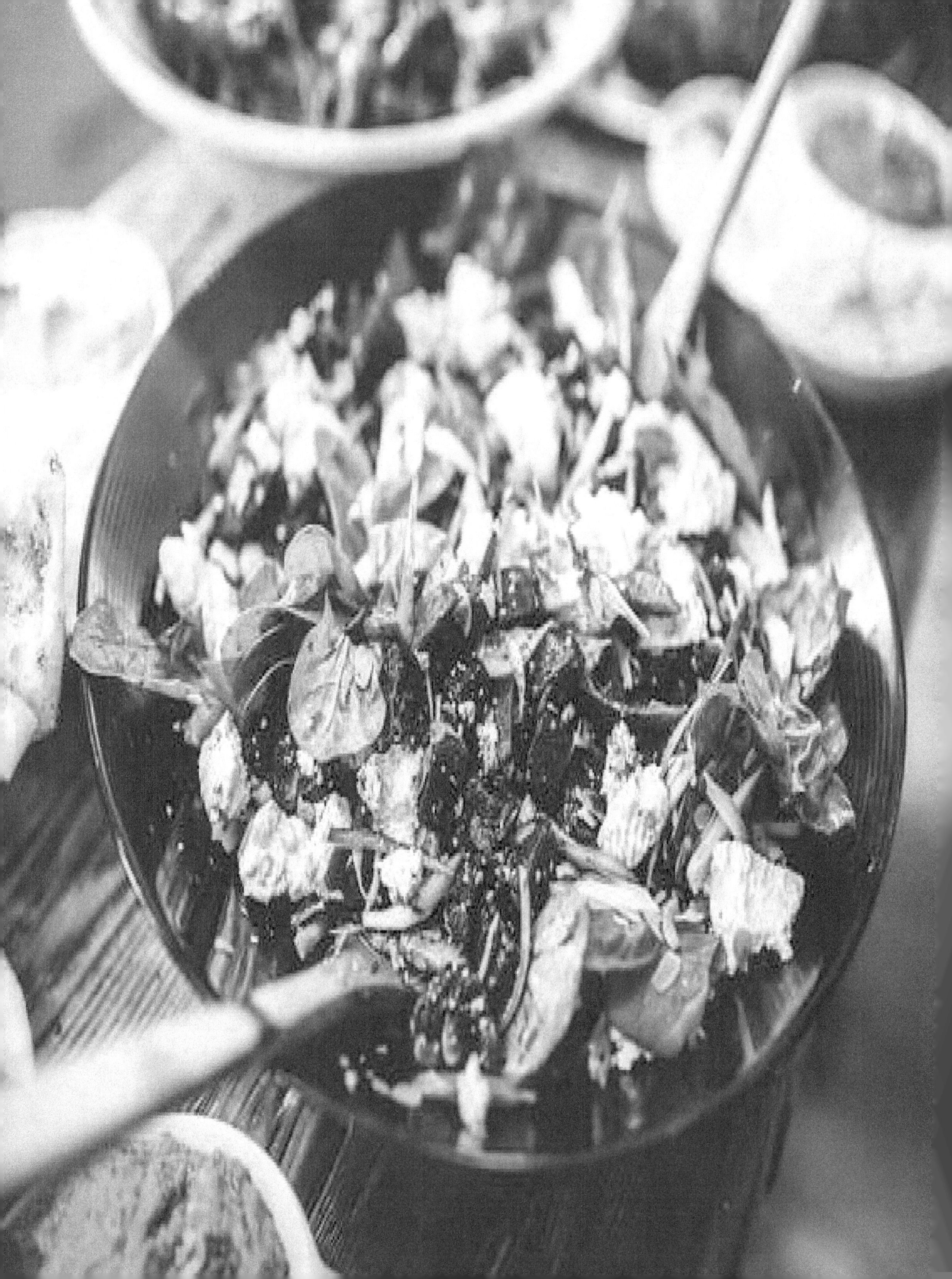

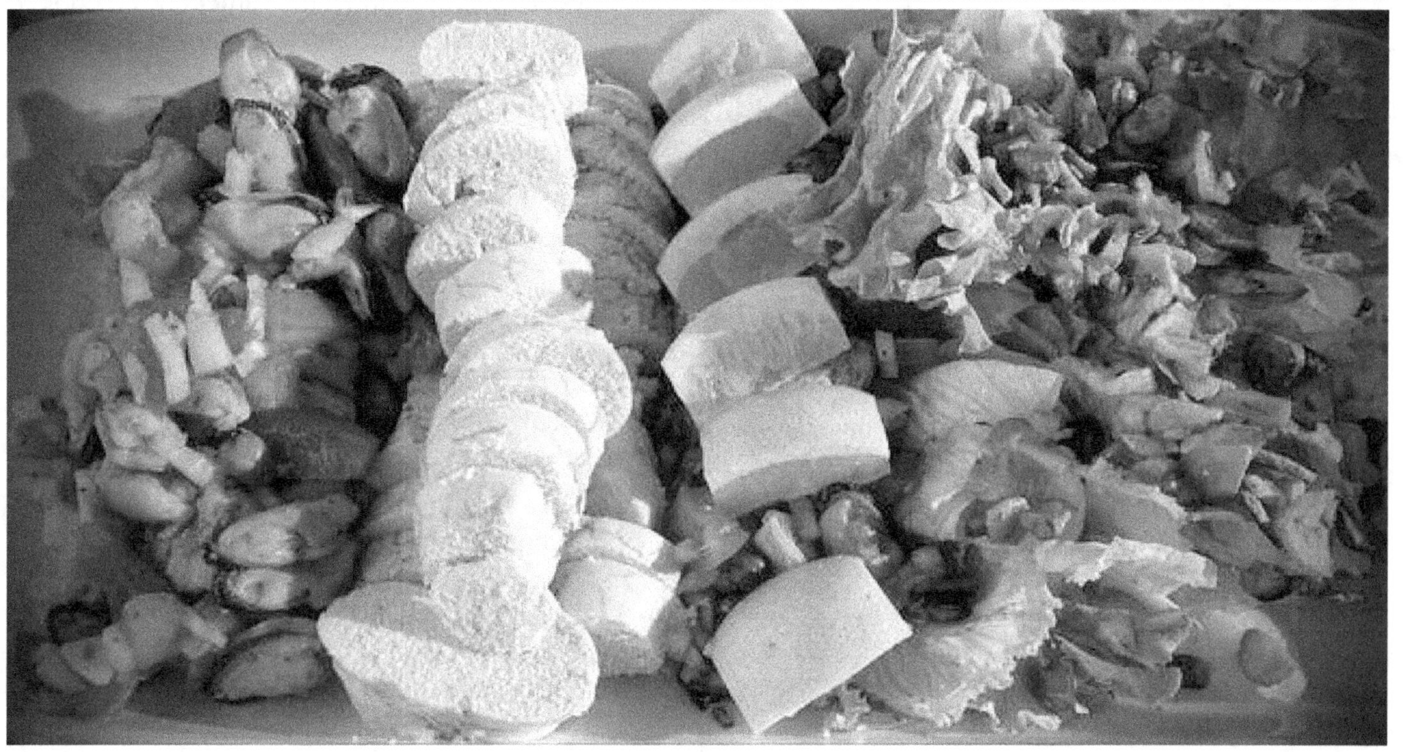

Baked Cod with Lemon and Herbs

⏱ **Prep Time:** 10 minutes | 🔍 **Cooking Time:** 15 minutes | 🍽 Servings: 2

🛒 **Ingredients:**

- 2 cod fillets
- 1 lemon, sliced
- 2 tablespoons olive oil
- 1 teaspoon dried thyme
- 1 teaspoon dried rosemary
- Salt and pepper to taste

📋 **Instructions:**

1. Preheat the oven to 400°F (200°C).
2. Place the cod fillets in a baking dish.
3. Drizzle olive oil over the fillets and sprinkle with thyme, rosemary, salt, and pepper.
4. Top with lemon slices.
5. Bake for 15 minutes or until the fish is opaque and flakes easily with a fork.
6. Serve immediately.

🍲 **Nutritional Information:** Calories: 220 | Protein: 24g | Carbs: 3g | Fat: 12g | Fiber: 1g

Chicken and Vegetable Skewers

⏱ **Prep Time:** 15 minutes | 🔍 **Cooking Time:** 15 minutes | 🍽 **Servings:** 4

🛒 **Ingredients:**

- 2 boneless, skinless chicken breasts, cut into cubes
- 1 red bell pepper, cut into chunks
- 1 yellow bell pepper, cut into chunks
- 1 zucchini, sliced
- 1 red onion, cut into chunks
- 2 tablespoons olive oil
- 2 tablespoons lemon juice
- 1 teaspoon dried oregano
- Salt and pepper to taste

1. Preheat the grill to medium-high heat.
2. In a large bowl, combine olive oil, lemon juice, oregano, salt, and pepper.
3. Add chicken and vegetables to the bowl, tossing to coat.
4. Thread chicken and vegetables onto skewers.
5. Grill for 10-15 minutes, turning occasionally, until the chicken is cooked through and vegetables are tender.
6. Serve immediately.

Nutritional Information: Calories: 300 | Protein: 25g | Carbs: 10g | Fat: 18g | Fiber: 3g

Grilled Eggplant and Tomato Stack

Prep Time: 10 minutes | **Cooking Time:** 15 minutes | Servings: 2

Ingredients:

- 1 large eggplant, sliced into rounds
- 2 large tomatoes, sliced
- 1/4 cup fresh basil leaves
- 2 tablespoons balsamic vinegar
- 2 tablespoons olive oil
- Salt and pepper to taste

Instructions:

1. Preheat the grill to medium heat.
2. Brush eggplant slices with olive oil and season with salt and pepper.
3. Grill eggplant slices for 5-7 minutes on each side until tender and slightly charred.
4. On a serving plate, stack grilled eggplant and tomato slices, layering with fresh basil leaves.
5. Drizzle with balsamic vinegar and additional olive oil if desired.
6. Serve immediately.

Nutritional Information: Calories: 150 | Protein: 2g | Carbs: 15g | Fat: 10g | Fiber: 5g

Spinach and Mushroom Stuffed Chicken Breast

Prep Time: 15 minutes | **Cooking Time:** 30 minutes | Servings: 2

Ingredients:

- 2 boneless, skinless chicken breasts
- 1 cup fresh spinach, chopped
- 1/2 cup mushrooms, chopped
- 1/4 cup feta cheese, crumbled
- 2 tablespoons olive oil
- Salt and pepper to taste

Instructions:

1. Preheat the oven to 375°F (190°C).
2. In a skillet, heat 1 tablespoon of olive oil over medium heat. Add mushrooms and cook until soft, about 5 minutes.
3. Add spinach to the skillet and cook until wilted, about 2 minutes.
4. Remove from heat and stir in feta cheese.
5. Cut a pocket into each chicken breast and stuff with the spinach mixture.
6. Secure with toothpicks if necessary.
7. Heat the remaining olive oil in an oven-safe skillet over medium-high heat. Sear the chicken breasts for 2-3 minutes on each side until golden brown.
8. Transfer the skillet to the preheated oven and bake for 20 minutes or until the chicken is cooked through.
9. Serve immediately.

Nutritional Information: Calories: 350 | Protein: 35g | Carbs: 5g | Fat: 20g | Fiber: 2g

Brown Rice and Lentil Pilaf

⏱ Prep Time: 10 minutes | **🔍 Cooking Time:** 40 minutes | **🍽 Servings:** 4

🛒 Ingredients:

- 1 cup brown rice
- 1/2 cup lentils, rinsed
- 1 onion, diced
- 2 garlic cloves, minced
- 3 cups vegetable broth
- 2 tablespoons olive oil
- 1 teaspoon cumin
- Salt and pepper to taste

📋 Instructions:

1. Heat olive oil in a large pot over medium heat.
2. Add onion and garlic, cooking until soft, about 5 minutes.
3. Stir in brown rice and cumin, cooking for 2 minutes.
4. Add lentils and vegetable broth. Bring to a boil.
5. Reduce heat, cover, and simmer for 35-40 minutes or until rice and lentils are tender.
6. Season with salt and pepper to taste.
7. Serve immediately.

🍱 Nutritional Information: Calories: 250 | Protein: 8g | Carbs: 45g | Fat: 6g | Fiber: 8g

Broiled Tilapia with Steamed Broccoli

⏱ Prep Time: 10 minutes | **🔍 Cooking Time:** 15 minutes | **🍽 Servings:** 2

🛒 Ingredients:

- 2 tilapia fillets
- 1 lemon, sliced
- 1 tablespoon olive oil
- 1 teaspoon paprika
- 2 cups broccoli florets
- Salt and pepper to taste

📋 Instructions:

1. Preheat the broiler.
2. Place the tilapia fillets on a baking sheet lined with foil.
3. Drizzle with olive oil and sprinkle with paprika, salt, and pepper.
4. Top with lemon slices.
5. Broil for 10-12 minutes or until the fish is cooked through and flakes easily with a fork.
6. While the fish is broiling, steam the broccoli florets until tender, about 5 minutes.
7. Serve the tilapia with steamed broccoli.

🍱 Nutritional Information: Calories: 220 | Protein: 28g | Carbs: 8g | Fat: 9g | Fiber: 4g

Quinoa-Stuffed Bell Peppers

⏱ Prep Time: 15 minutes | **🔍 Cooking Time:** 25 minutes | **🍽 Servings:** 4

🛒 Ingredients:

- 4 large bell peppers
- 1 cup cooked quinoa
- 1 can (15 oz) black beans, rinsed and drained
- 1 cup corn kernels (fresh or frozen)
- 1/2 cup diced tomatoes
- 1/4 cup chopped cilantro
- 2 tablespoons lime juice
- 1 teaspoon cumin
- Salt and pepper to taste

📋 Instructions:

1. Preheat the oven to 375°F (190°C).

2. Cut the tops off the bell peppers and remove the seeds and membranes.
3. In a large bowl, combine cooked quinoa, black beans, corn, diced tomatoes, cilantro, lime juice, cumin, salt, and pepper.
4. Stuff the bell peppers with the quinoa mixture.
5. Place the stuffed peppers in a baking dish and cover with foil.
6. Bake for 20 minutes, then remove the foil and bake for an additional 5 minutes.
7. Serve warm.

Nutritional Information: Calories: 220 | Protein: 8g | Carbs: 35g | Fat: 5g | Fiber: 8g

Roasted Turkey Breast with Brussels Sprouts

Prep Time: 10 minutes | **Cooking Time:** 40 minutes | **Servings:** 4

Ingredients:

- 1 boneless turkey breast
- 1 pound Brussels sprouts, halved
- 3 tablespoons olive oil
- 2 tablespoons lemon juice
- 1 teaspoon dried thyme
- Salt and pepper to taste

Instructions:

1. Preheat the oven to 375°F (190°C).
2. In a small bowl, mix 2 tablespoons of olive oil, lemon juice, thyme, salt, and pepper. Rub the mixture over the turkey breast.
3. Place the turkey breast on a baking sheet and roast for 30-40 minutes, or until the internal temperature reaches 165°F (74°C).
4. While the turkey is roasting, toss the Brussels sprouts with the remaining olive oil, salt, and pepper.
5. Add the Brussels sprouts to the baking sheet during the last 20 minutes of roasting.
6. Let the turkey rest for a few minutes before slicing.
7. Serve the turkey slices with roasted Brussels sprouts.

Nutritional Information: Calories: 300 | Protein: 35g | Carbs: 10g | Fat: 15g | Fiber: 5g

Garlic Shrimp with Zucchini Noodles

Prep Time: 10 minutes | **Cooking Time:** 10 minutes | **Servings:** 2

Ingredients:

- 1 pound shrimp, peeled and deveined
- 2 medium zucchinis, spiralized
- 3 garlic cloves, minced
- 2 tablespoons olive oil
- 1/4 teaspoon red pepper flakes
- 1 tablespoon lemon juice
- Salt and pepper to taste
- Fresh parsley, chopped (for garnish)

Instructions:

1. Heat olive oil in a large skillet over medium heat.
2. Add garlic and red pepper flakes, cooking for 1 minute until fragrant.
3. Add shrimp to the skillet and cook for 2-3 minutes on each side until pink and opaque.
4. Remove shrimp from the skillet and set aside.
5. In the same skillet, add zucchini noodles and cook for 2-3 minutes until tender.
6. Return shrimp to the skillet and toss with zucchini noodles.
7. Add lemon juice and season with salt and pepper.
8. Garnish with fresh parsley and serve immediately.

Nutritional Information: Calories: 250 | Protein: 30g | Carbs: 10g | Fat: 10g | Fiber: 3g

Herb-Rubbed Pork Tenderloin with Roasted Vegetables

Prep Time: 15 minutes | **Cooking Time:** 25 minutes | **Servings:** 4

Ingredients:

- 1 pork tenderloin
- 1 teaspoon dried rosemary
- 1 teaspoon dried thyme
- 1 teaspoon garlic powder
- 2 tablespoons olive oil
- Salt and pepper to taste
- 2 cups mixed vegetables (carrots, bell peppers, onions), chopped

Instructions:

1. Preheat the oven to 400°F (200°C).
2. In a small bowl, mix rosemary, thyme, garlic powder, salt, and pepper.
3. Rub the herb mixture all over the pork tenderloin.
4. Heat 1 tablespoon of olive oil in a large skillet over medium-high heat. Sear the pork tenderloin on all sides until browned, about 5 minutes.
5. Place the pork tenderloin on a baking sheet lined with foil.
6. Toss the mixed vegetables with the remaining olive oil, salt, and pepper, and spread around the pork on the baking sheet.
7. Roast for 20-25 minutes, or until the internal temperature of the pork reaches 145°F (63°C).
8. Let the pork rest for a few minutes before slicing.
9. Serve the pork slices with roasted vegetables.

Nutritional Information: Calories: 320 | Protein: 30g | Carbs: 15g | Fat: 15g | Fiber: 5g

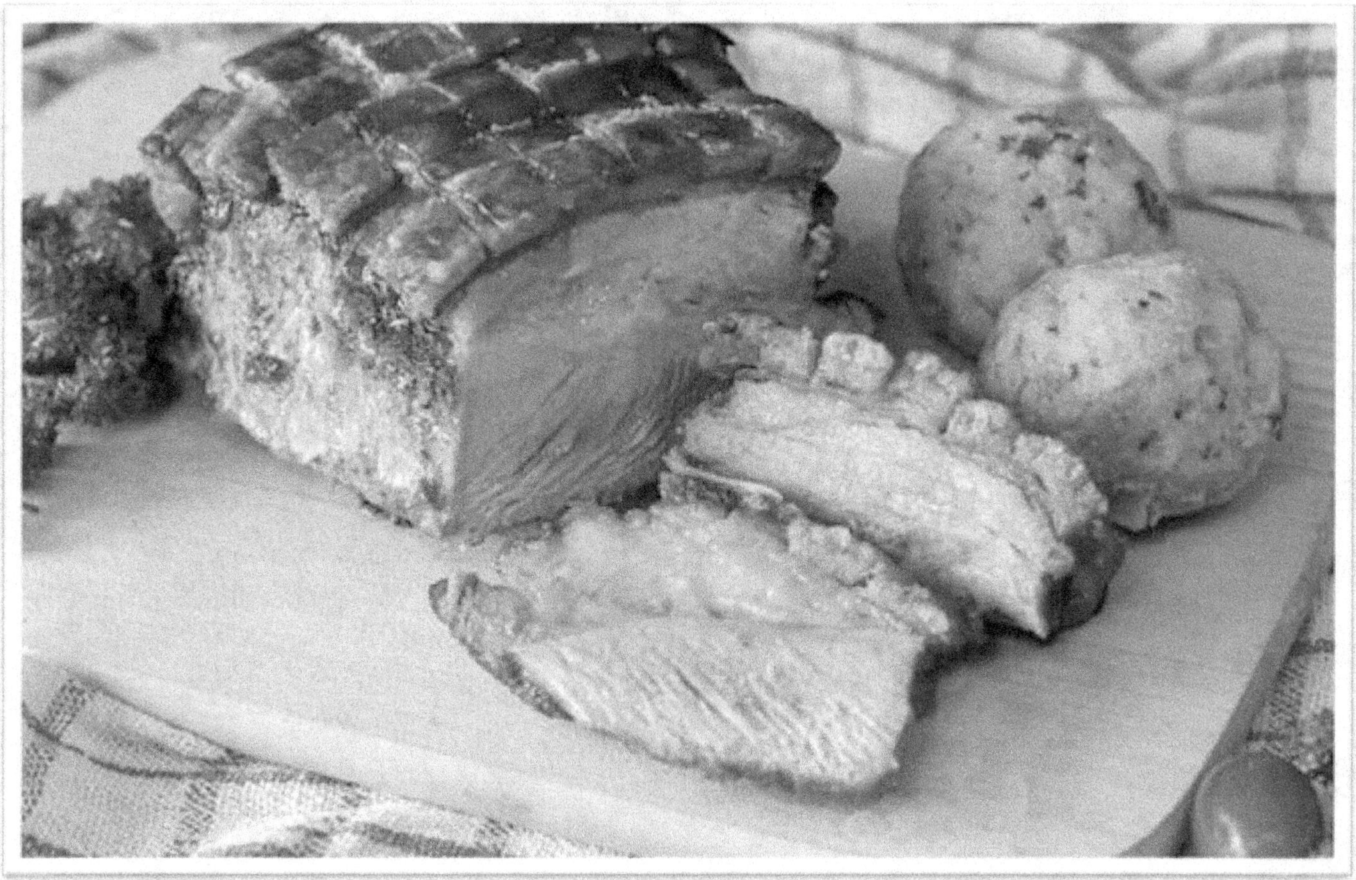

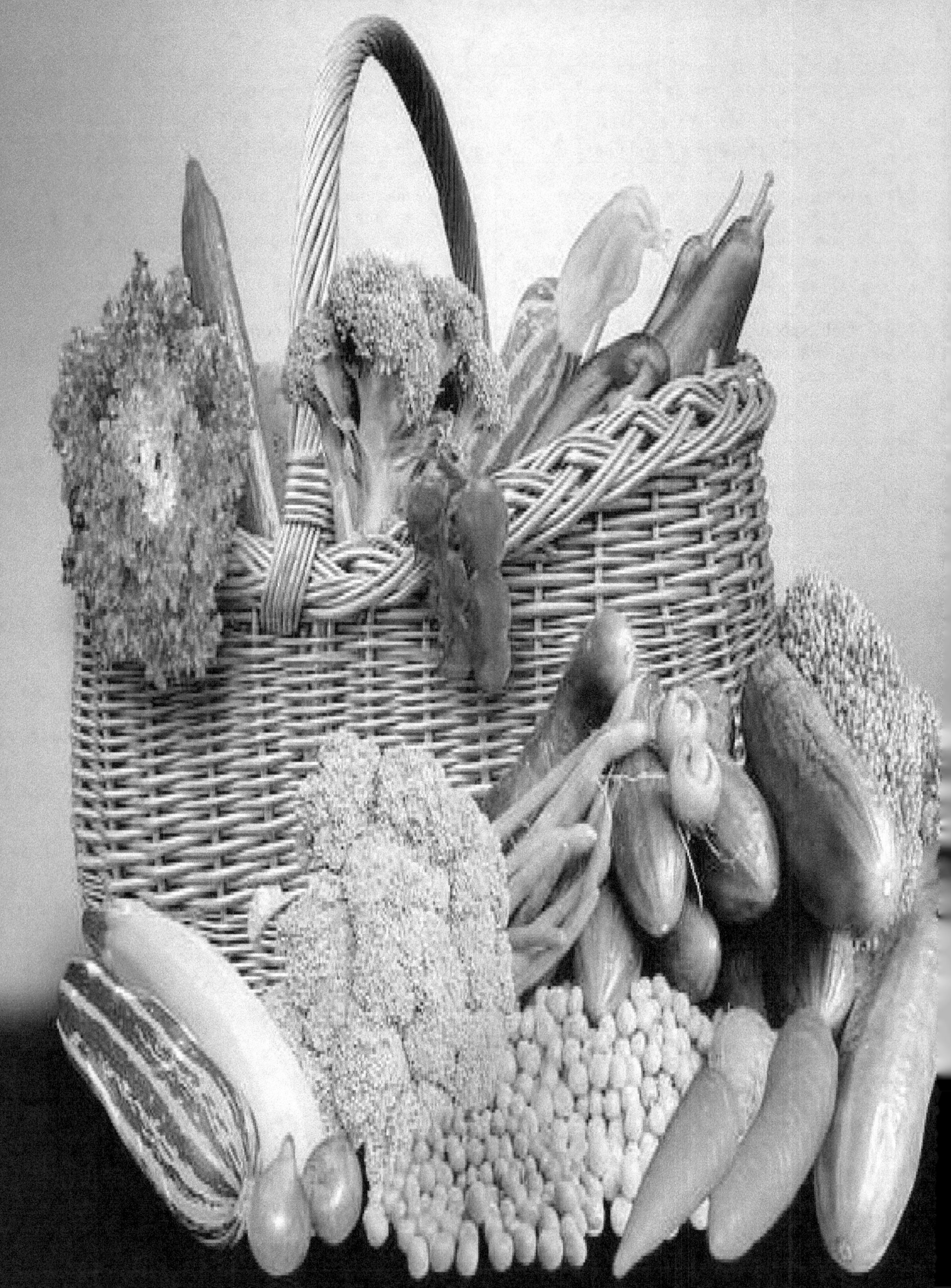

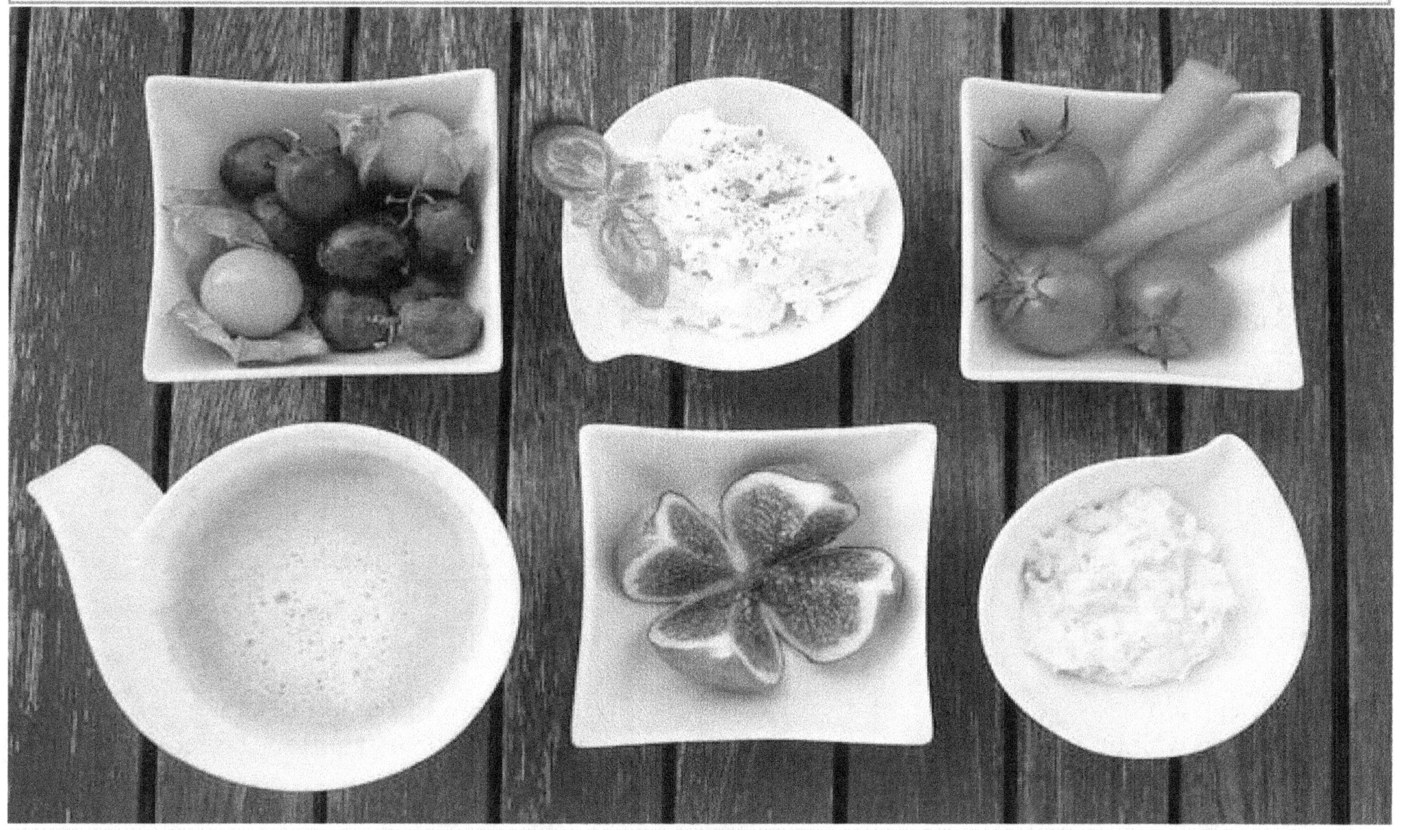

Carrot and Hummus Cups

Prep Time: 5 minutes | **Cooking Time:** 0 minutes | Servings: 2

Ingredients:

- 2 large carrots, cut into sticks
- 1/2 cup hummus

Instructions:

1. Cut the carrots into sticks.
2. Divide the hummus into small cups or bowls.
3. Serve the carrot sticks with the hummus for dipping.

Nutritional Information: Calories: 150 | Protein: 5g | Carbs: 18g | Fat: 8g | Fiber: 6g

Apple Slices with Almond Butter

Prep Time: 5 minutes | **Cooking Time:** 0 minutes | Servings: 2

Ingredients:

- 1 large apple, sliced
- 2 tablespoons almond butter

Instructions:

1. Core and slice the apple.
2. Serve the apple slices with almond butter for dipping.

Nutritional Information: Calories: 200 | Protein: 4g | Carbs: 26g | Fat: 10g | Fiber: 6g

Cucumber and Tomato Salad

⏱**Prep Time:** 10 minutes | 🔍**Cooking Time:** 0 minutes | 🍽🍽🍽**Servings:** 2

🛒 **Ingredients:**

- 1 cucumber, sliced
- 1 cup cherry tomatoes, halved
- 1 tablespoon olive oil
- 1 tablespoon red wine vinegar
- Salt and pepper to taste

📋**Instructions:**

1. In a bowl, combine cucumber slices and cherry tomatoes.
2. Drizzle with olive oil and red wine vinegar.
3. Season with salt and pepper to taste.
4. Toss to combine and serve immediately.

🍲**Nutritional Information:** Calories: 100 | Protein: 2g | Carbs: 12g | Fat: 7g | Fiber: 3g

Mixed Nuts and Seeds Trail Mix

⏱**Prep Time:** 5 minutes | 🔍**Cooking Time:** 0 minutes | 🍽**Servings:** 4

🛒 **Ingredients:**

- 1/2 cup almonds
- 1/2 cup walnuts
- 1/4 cup pumpkin seeds
- 1/4 cup sunflower seeds
- 1/4 cup dried cranberries

📋**Instructions:**

1. In a bowl, combine almonds, walnuts, pumpkin seeds, sunflower seeds, and dried cranberries.
2. Mix well and divide into portions.
3. Serve immediately or store in an airtight container for later.

🍲**Nutritional Information:** Calories: 250 | Protein: 6g | Carbs: 16g | Fat: 20g | Fiber: 5g

Edamame with Sea Salt

⏱**Prep Time:** 5 minutes | 🔍**Cooking Time:** 5 minutes | 🍽**Servings:** 2

🛒 **Ingredients:**

- 1 cup edamame (in the pod)
- Sea salt to taste

📋**Instructions:**

1. Boil or steam the edamame for about 5 minutes until tender.
2. Drain and sprinkle with sea salt.
3. Serve immediately.

🍲**Nutritional Information:** Calories: 120 | Protein: 10g | Carbs: 10g | Fat: 4g | Fiber: 5g

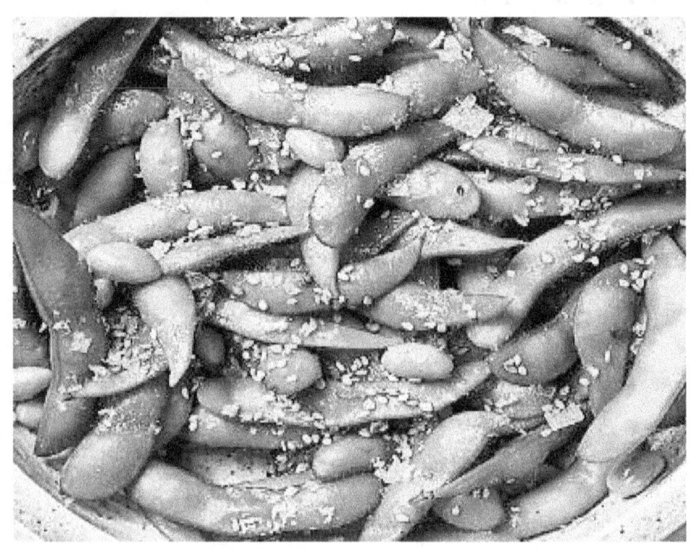

Cottage Cheese with Pineapple

⏱ **Prep Time:** 5 minutes | 🔍 **Cooking Time:** 0 minutes | 🍽 Servings: 2

🛒 **Ingredients:**

- 1 cup cottage cheese
- 1/2 cup pineapple chunks (fresh or canned in juice)

📋 **Instructions:**

1. In a bowl, combine cottage cheese and pineapple chunks.
2. Mix well and serve immediately.

🥗 **Nutritional Information:** Calories: 150 | Protein: 14g | Carbs: 15g | Fat: 4g | Fiber: 2g

Bell Pepper Strips with Guacamole

⏱ **Prep Time:** 5 minutes | 🔍 **Cooking Time:** 0 minutes | 🍽 Servings: 2

🛒 **Ingredients:**

- 2 bell peppers (any color), cut into strips
- 1/2 cup guacamole

📋 **Instructions:**

1. Cut the bell peppers into strips.
2. Serve the bell pepper strips with guacamole for dipping.

🥗 **Nutritional Information:** Calories: 150 | Protein: 2g | Carbs: 18g | Fat: 10g | Fiber: 6g

Greek Yogurt with Cucumber and Dill

⏱ **Prep Time:** 5 minutes | 🔍 **Cooking Time:** 0 minutes | 🍽 Servings: 2

🛒 **Ingredients:**

- 1 cup Greek yogurt
- 1/2 cucumber, grated
- 1 tablespoon fresh dill, chopped
- Salt and pepper to taste

📋 **Instructions:**

1. In a bowl, combine Greek yogurt, grated cucumber, and chopped dill.
2. Season with salt and pepper to taste.
3. Mix well and serve immediately.

🥗 **Nutritional Information:** Calories: 100 | Protein: 10g | Carbs: 8g | Fat: 4g | Fiber: 1g

Almonds and Dried Apricots

⏱ **Prep Time:** 2 minutes | 🔍 **Cooking Time:** 0 minutes | 🍽 Servings: 2

🛒 **Ingredients:**

- 1/4 cup almonds
- 1/4 cup dried apricots

📋 **Instructions:**

1. In a bowl, combine almonds and dried apricots.
2. Mix well and serve immediately or store in an airtight container for later.

🥗 **Nutritional Information:** Calories: 200 | Protein: 4g | Carbs: 30g | Fat: 10g | Fiber: 5g

Celery Sticks with Peanut Butter

⏱ Prep Time: 5 minutes | **🔍 Cooking Time:** 0 minutes | **🍴 Servings: 2**

🛒 Ingredients:

- 4 celery sticks
- 2 tablespoons peanut butter

📋 Instructions:

1. Wash and cut the celery sticks.
2. Spread peanut butter into the grooves of the celery sticks.
3. Serve immediately.

🥗 **Nutritional Information:** Calories: 150 | Protein: 5g | Carbs: 10g | Fat: 12g | Fiber: 4g

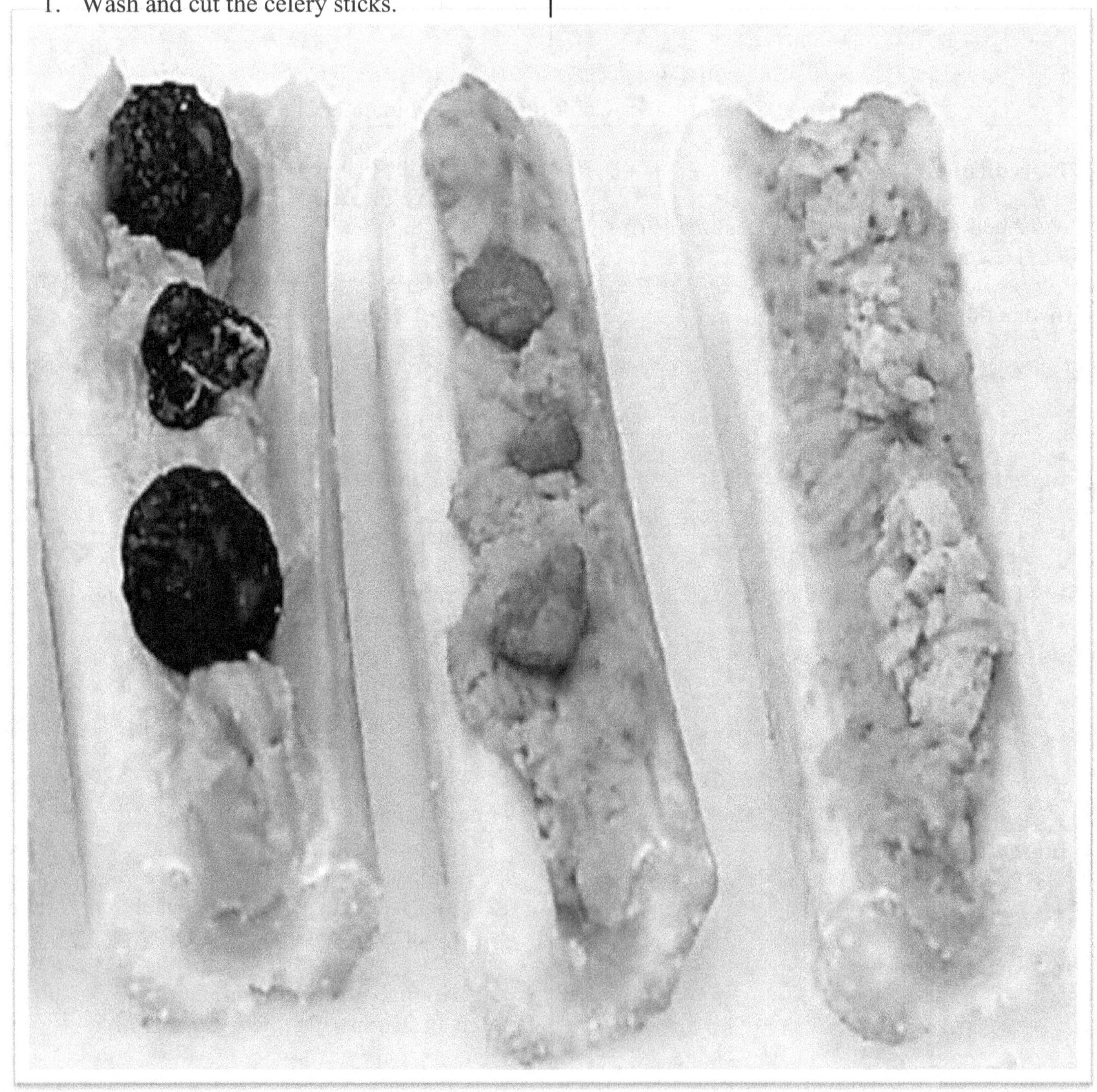

Spinach and Berry Smoothie

⏱ **Prep Time:** 5 minutes | 🔍 **Cooking Time:** 0 minutes | 🍽 Servings: 2

🛒 **Ingredients:**

- 1 cup fresh spinach
- 1 cup mixed berries (strawberries, blueberries, raspberries)
- 1 banana
- 1 cup unsweetened almond milk
- 1 tablespoon chia seeds
- 1 teaspoon honey (optional)

📋 **Instructions:**

1. Combine spinach, mixed berries, banana, almond milk, and chia seeds in a blender.
2. Blend until smooth.
3. Taste and add honey if desired.
4. Pour into glasses and serve immediately.

🥗 **Nutritional Information:** Calories: 180 | Protein: 3g | Carbs: 36g | Fat: 4g | Fiber: 8g

Green Tea with Lemon

⏱ **Prep Time:** 2 minutes | 🔍 **Cooking Time:** 5 minutes | 🍽 Servings: 2

🛒 **Ingredients:**

- 2 green tea bags
- 2 cups hot water
- 1 lemon, sliced
- Honey (optional)

📋 **Instructions:**

1. Steep the green tea bags in hot water for 3-5 minutes.
2. Remove the tea bags and add lemon slices.
3. Sweeten with honey if desired.
4. Serve hot.

🥗 **Nutritional Information:** Calories: 10 | Protein: 0g | Carbs: 3g | Fat: 0g | Fiber: 0g

Cucumber and Mint Infused Water

⏱ Prep Time: 5 minutes | **🔍 Cooking Time:** 0 minutes | **🍴 Servings:** 4

🛒 Ingredients:

- 1 cucumber, sliced
- 10 fresh mint leaves
- 1 liter water

📋 Instructions:

1. In a pitcher, combine cucumber slices and mint leaves.
2. Fill with water.
3. Refrigerate for at least 1 hour to allow flavors to infuse.
4. Serve chilled.

🍚 **Nutritional Information:** Calories: 0 | Protein: 0g | Carbs: 0g | Fat: 0g | Fiber: 0g

Berry and Almond Milk Smoothie

⏱ Prep Time: 5 minutes | **🔍 Cooking Time:** 0 minutes | **🍴 Servings:** 2

🛒 Ingredients:

- 1 cup mixed berries (strawberries, blueberries, raspberries)
- 1 banana
- 1 cup unsweetened almond milk
- 1 tablespoon flaxseed
- 1 teaspoon honey (optional)

📋 Instructions:

1. Combine mixed berries, banana, almond milk, and flaxseed in a blender.
2. Blend until smooth.
3. Taste and add honey if desired.
4. Pour into glasses and serve immediately.

🍚 **Nutritional Information:** Calories: 190 | Protein: 3g | Carbs: 40g | Fat: 4g | Fiber: 7g

Turmeric and Ginger Detox Drink

⏱ Prep Time: 5 minutes | **🔍 Cooking Time:** 0 minutes | **🍴 Servings:** 2

🛒 Ingredients:

- 2 cups water
- 1 teaspoon turmeric powder
- 1 teaspoon grated ginger
- 1 tablespoon lemon juice
- Honey (optional)

📋 Instructions:

1. In a pitcher, combine water, turmeric powder, grated ginger, and lemon juice.
2. Stir well and let sit for 5 minutes.
3. Sweeten with honey if desired.
4. Serve chilled or at room temperature.

🍚 **Nutritional Information:** Calories: 15 | Protein: 0g | Carbs: 4g | Fat: 0g | Fiber: 0g

Kale and Pineapple Smoothie

⏱ Prep Time: 5 minutes | **🔍 Cooking Time:** 0 minutes | **🍴 Servings:** 2

🛒 Ingredients:

- 1 cup kale leaves, chopped
- 1 cup pineapple chunks
- 1 banana
- 1 cup coconut water

- 1 tablespoon chia seeds

📋 **Instructions:**

1. Combine kale, pineapple, banana, coconut water, and chia seeds in a blender.
2. Blend until smooth.
3. Pour into glasses and serve immediately.

🍱 **Nutritional Information:** Calories: 170 | Protein: 2g | Carbs: 40g | Fat: 1g | Fiber: 6g

Lemon and Cucumber Detox Water

⏱ **Prep Time:** 5 minutes | 🔍 **Cooking Time:** 0 minutes | 🍽 **Servings:** 4

🛒 **Ingredients:**

- 1 lemon, sliced
- 1 cucumber, sliced
- 1 liter water

📋 **Instructions:**

1. In a pitcher, combine lemon slices and cucumber slices.
2. Fill with water.
3. Refrigerate for at least 1 hour to allow flavors to infuse.
4. Serve chilled.

🍱 **Nutritional Information:** Calories: 0 | Protein: 0g | Carbs: 0g | Fat: 0g | Fiber: 0g

Blueberry and Spinach Smoothie

⏱ **Prep Time:** 5 minutes | 🔍 **Cooking Time:** 0 minutes | 🍽 **Servings:** 2

🛒 **Ingredients:**

- 1 cup fresh spinach
- 1 cup blueberries
- 1 banana
- 1 cup unsweetened almond milk
- 1 tablespoon chia seeds

📋 **Instructions:**

1. Combine spinach, blueberries, banana, almond milk, and chia seeds in a blender.
2. Blend until smooth.
3. Pour into glasses and serve immediately.

🍱 **Nutritional Information:** Calories: 170 | Protein: 3g | Carbs: 35g | Fat: 4g | Fiber: 7g

Apple Cider Vinegar Tonic

⏱ **Prep Time:** 2 minutes | 🔍 **Cooking Time:** 0 minutes | 🍽 **Servings:** 2

🛒 **Ingredients:**

- 2 tablespoons apple cider vinegar
- 2 cups water
- 1 tablespoon lemon juice
- 1 teaspoon honey (optional)
- Pinch of cayenne pepper (optional)

📋 **Instructions:**

1. In a pitcher, combine apple cider vinegar, water, lemon juice, honey, and cayenne pepper if using.
2. Stir well to mix.
3. Serve chilled or at room temperature.

🍱 **Nutritional Information:** Calories: 10 | Protein: 0g | Carbs: 3g | Fat: 0g | Fiber: 0g

Beet and Carrot Juice

🛒 Ingredients:

- 2 medium beets, peeled and chopped
- 2 large carrots, peeled and chopped
- 1 apple, cored and chopped
- 1 tablespoon lemon juice
- 1 cup water

📋 Instructions:

1. In a blender, combine beets, carrots, apple, lemon juice, and water.
2. Blend until smooth.
3. Strain through a fine mesh sieve or cheesecloth into a pitcher.
4. Serve immediately.

🥗 **Nutritional Information:** Calories: 120 | Protein: 2g | Carbs: 30g | Fat: 0g | Fiber: 6g

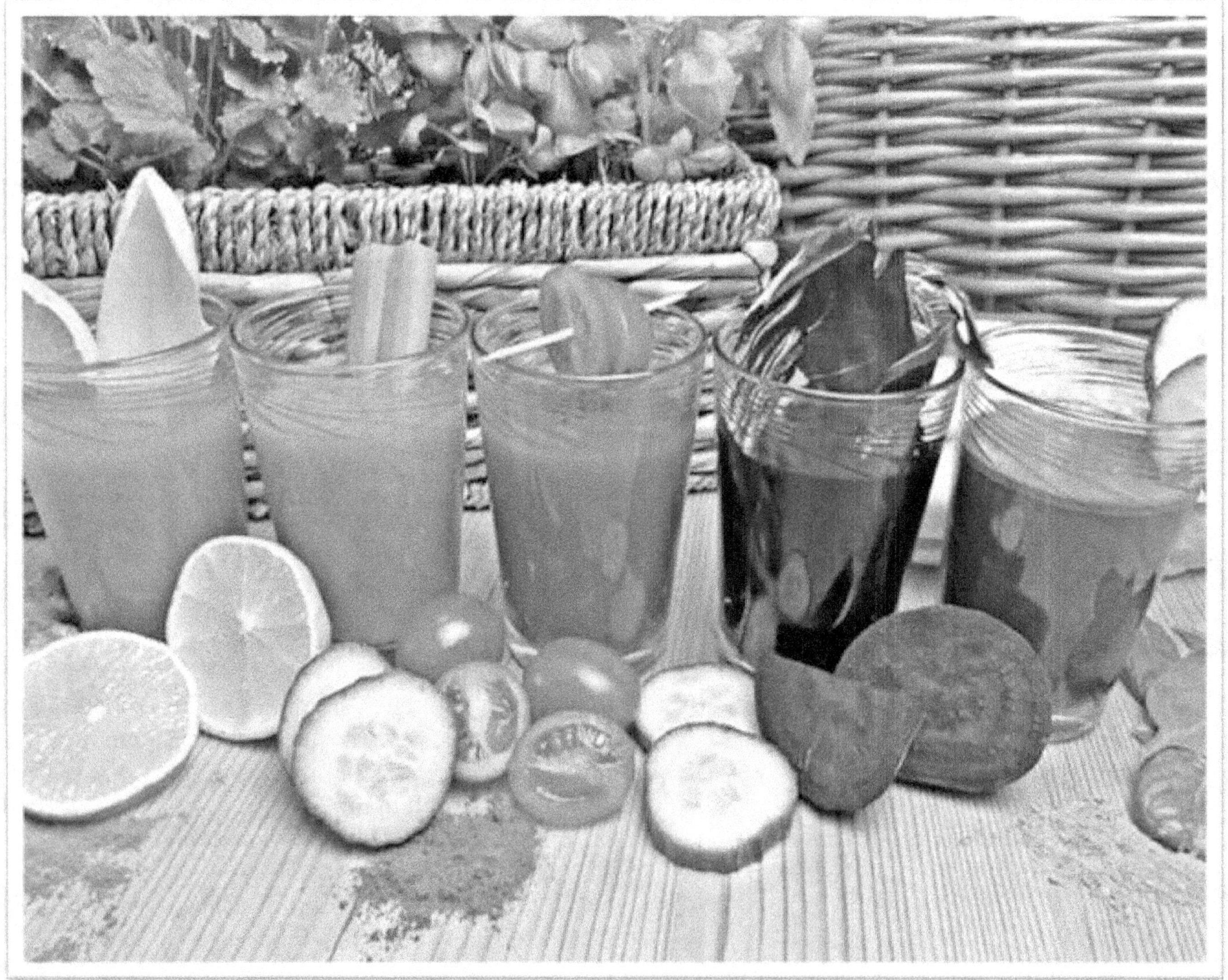

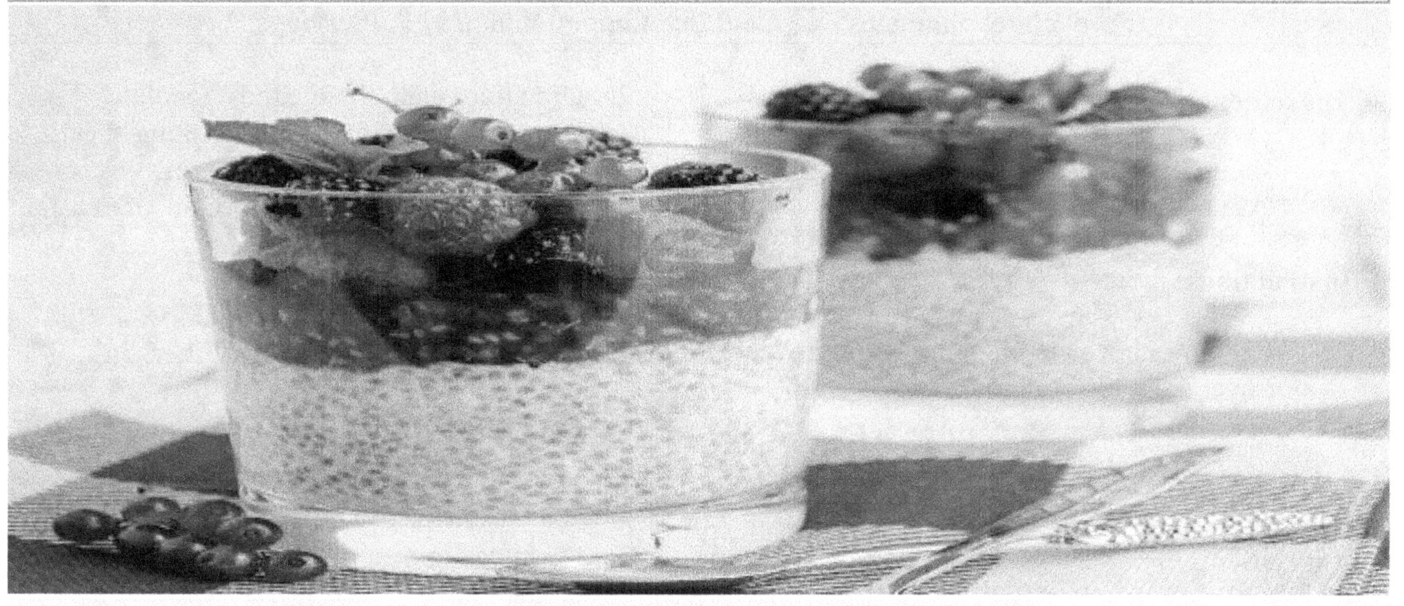

Chia Seed Pudding with Almond Milk

⏱ Prep Time: 5 minutes | **🔍 Cooking Time:** 0 minutes | **🍽 Servings:** 2

🛒 Ingredients:

- 1/4 cup chia seeds
- 1 cup unsweetened almond milk
- 1 tablespoon honey
- 1/2 teaspoon vanilla extract
- Fresh berries for topping

📋 Instructions:

1. In a bowl, whisk together chia seeds, almond milk, honey, and vanilla extract.
2. Cover and refrigerate for at least 4 hours or overnight.
3. Stir the pudding and divide into bowls.
4. Top with fresh berries before serving.

🍱 **Nutritional Information:** Calories: 200 | Protein: 4g | Carbs: 30g | Fat: 9g | Fiber: 10g

Fresh Berry Salad

⏱ Prep Time: 10 minutes | **🔍 Cooking Time:** 0 minutes | **🍽 Servings:** 2

🛒 Ingredients:

- 1 cup strawberries, hulled and sliced
- 1 cup blueberries
- 1 cup raspberries
- 1 tablespoon fresh mint, chopped
- 1 tablespoon honey (optional)
- 1 teaspoon lemon juice

📋 Instructions:

1. In a large bowl, combine strawberries, blueberries, raspberries, and chopped mint.
2. Drizzle with honey and lemon juice if desired.
3. Toss gently to combine.
4. Serve immediately.

🍱 **Nutritional Information:** Calories: 100 | Protein: 1g | Carbs: 25g | Fat: 0g | Fiber: 8g

Dark Chocolate and Almond Bites

⏱ **Prep Time:** 5 minutes | 🔍 **Cooking Time:** 0 minutes | 🍽 Servings: 2

🛒 **Ingredients:**

- 1/4 cup dark chocolate chips
- 1/4 cup almonds

📋 **Instructions:**

1. Melt dark chocolate chips in the microwave or over a double boiler.
2. Dip almonds in the melted chocolate.
3. Place on a parchment-lined baking sheet.
4. Refrigerate until chocolate is set.
5. Serve immediately or store in an airtight container.

🥗 **Nutritional Information:** Calories: 200 | Protein: 4g | Carbs: 18g | Fat: 14g | Fiber: 5g

Grilled Pineapple with Cinnamon

⏱ **Prep Time:** 5 minutes | 🔍 **Cooking Time:** 10 minutes | 🍽 Servings: 2

🛒 **Ingredients:**

- 1 pineapple, peeled and sliced
- 1 teaspoon ground cinnamon

📋 **Instructions:**

1. Preheat the grill to medium heat.
2. Sprinkle pineapple slices with ground cinnamon.
3. Grill pineapple slices for 3-5 minutes on each side until caramelized.
4. Serve warm.

🥗 **Nutritional Information:** Calories: 100 | Protein: 1g | Carbs: 25g | Fat: 0g | Fiber: 2g

Baked Apples with Oats and Honey

⏱ **Prep Time:** 10 minutes | 🔍 **Cooking Time:** 25 minutes | 🍽 Servings: 2

🛒 **Ingredients:**

- 2 apples, cored
- 1/4 cup rolled oats
- 1 tablespoon honey
- 1/2 teaspoon ground cinnamon
- 1 tablespoon butter

📋 **Instructions:**

1. Preheat the oven to 375°F (190°C).
2. In a small bowl, combine rolled oats, honey, ground cinnamon, and butter.
3. Stuff the mixture into the cored apples.
4. Place the apples in a baking dish and bake for 25 minutes or until tender.
5. Serve warm.

🥗 **Nutritional Information:** Calories: 200 | Protein: 2g | Carbs: 40g | Fat: 6g | Fiber: 6g

Avocado Chocolate Mousse

⏱ **Prep Time:** 5 minutes | 🔍 **Cooking Time:** 0 minutes | 🍽 Servings: 2

🛒 **Ingredients:**

- 1 ripe avocado
- 1/4 cup cocoa powder
- 1/4 cup almond milk
- 2 tablespoons honey
- 1 teaspoon vanilla extract

Instructions:

1. In a blender, combine avocado, cocoa powder, almond milk, honey, and vanilla extract.
2. Blend until smooth and creamy.

3. Divide into bowls and refrigerate for at least 30 minutes before serving.

Nutritional Information: Calories: 220 | Protein: 3g | Carbs: 26g | Fat: 14g | Fiber: 8g

Coconut Yogurt with Mango

Prep Time: 5 minutes | **Cooking Time:** 0 minutes | **Servings:** 2

Ingredients:

- 1 cup coconut yogurt
- 1 mango, peeled and diced
- 1 tablespoon shredded coconut

Instructions:

1. In a bowl, combine coconut yogurt and diced mango.
2. Sprinkle with shredded coconut.
3. Serve immediately.

Nutritional Information: Calories: 180 | Protein: 2g | Carbs: 30g | Fat: 7g | Fiber: 4g

Frozen Banana Bites

Prep Time: 10 minutes | **Cooking Time:** 0 minutes | **Servings:** 2

Ingredients:

- 2 bananas, sliced
- 1/4 cup dark chocolate chips
- 1 tablespoon coconut oil

Instructions:

1. Line a baking sheet with parchment paper.
2. Arrange banana slices on the baking sheet.

3. Melt dark chocolate chips and coconut oil in the microwave or over a double boiler.
4. Drizzle or dip banana slices in the melted chocolate.
5. Freeze for at least 2 hours until firm.
6. Serve frozen.

Nutritional Information: Calories: 150 | Protein: 1g | Carbs: 30g | Fat: 6g | Fiber: 3g

Almond Flour Brownies

Prep Time: 10 minutes | **Cooking Time:** 20 minutes | **Servings:** 4

Ingredients:

- 1 cup almond flour
- 1/4 cup cocoa powder
- 1/2 teaspoon baking soda
- 1/4 teaspoon salt
- 1/4 cup honey
- 2 eggs
- 1/4 cup coconut oil, melted
- 1 teaspoon vanilla extract

Instructions:

1. Preheat the oven to 350°F (175°C).
2. In a large bowl, mix almond flour, cocoa powder, baking soda, and salt.
3. In another bowl, whisk together honey, eggs, melted coconut oil, and vanilla extract.
4. Combine wet and dry ingredients, mixing well.
5. Pour the batter into a greased baking dish.

6. Bake for 20 minutes or until a toothpick inserted into the center comes out clean.
7. Let cool before slicing and serving.

🍰 **Nutritional Information:** Calories: 250 | Protein: 6g | Carbs: 20g | Fat: 18g | Fiber: 4g

Raspberry Chia Jam

⏱️ **Prep Time:** 5 minutes | 🔍 **Cooking Time:** 0 minutes | 🍽️ Servings: 2

🛒 **Ingredients:**

- 1 cup fresh raspberries
- 2 tablespoons chia seeds
- 1 tablespoon honey
- 1 teaspoon lemon juice

📋 **Instructions:**

1. In a bowl, mash the raspberries with a fork.
2. Stir in chia seeds, honey, and lemon juice.
3. Cover and refrigerate for at least 1 hour to thicken.
4. Serve as a spread or topping.

🍰 **Nutritional Information:** Calories: 50 | Protein: 1g | Carbs: 10g | Fat: 2g | Fiber: 5g

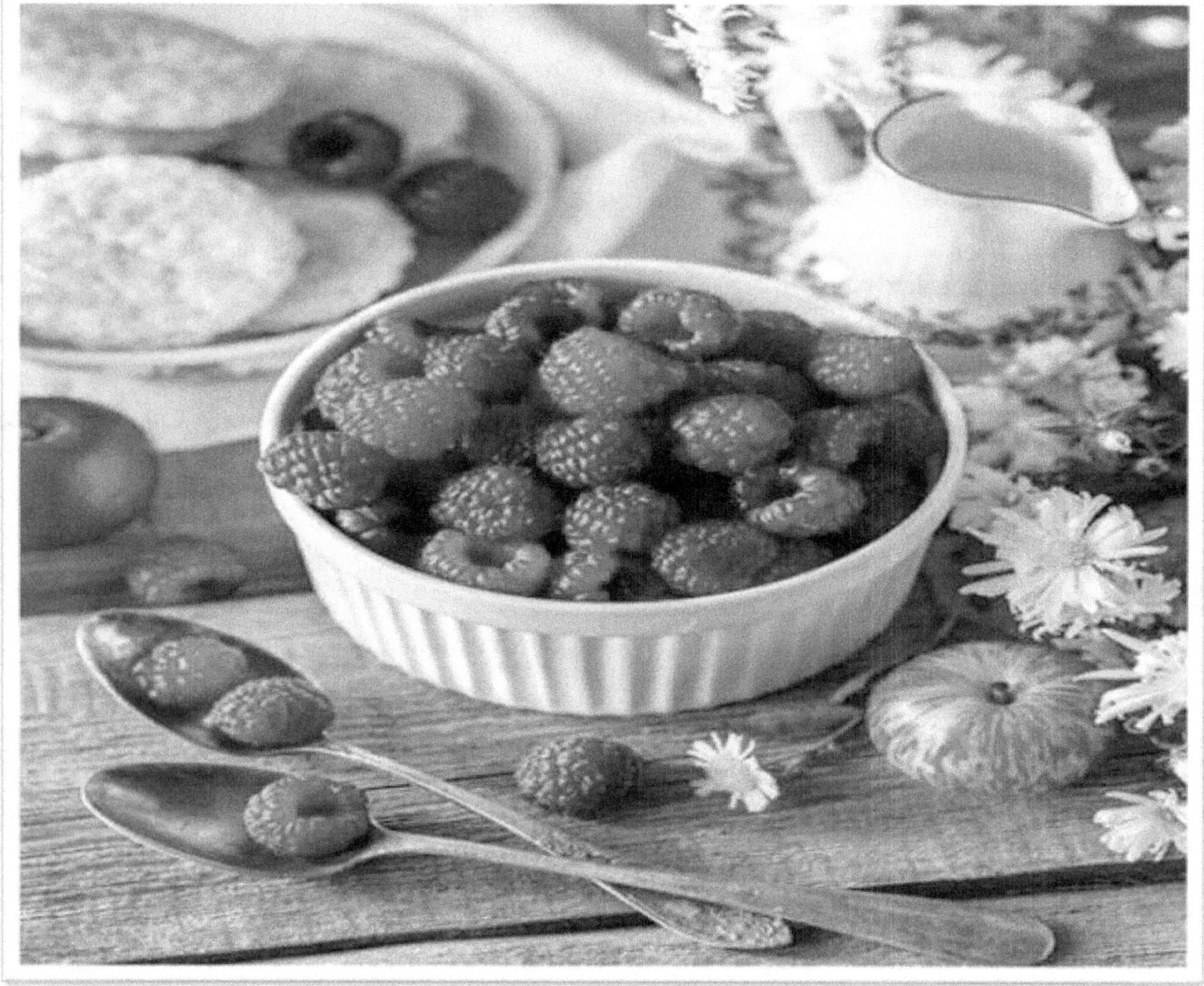

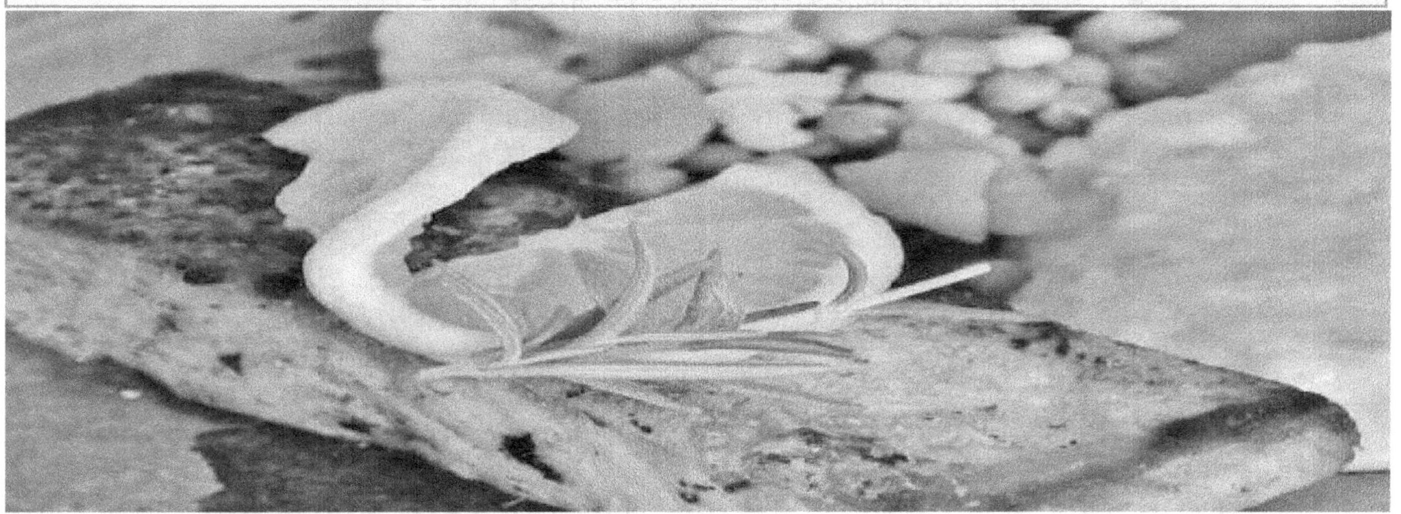

Baked Herb-Crusted Chicken

⏱ **Prep Time:** 10 minutes | 🔍 **Cooking Time:** 30 minutes | 🍽 **Servings:** 4

🛒 **Ingredients:**

- 4 boneless, skinless chicken breasts
- 1/2 cup breadcrumbs
- 1/4 cup grated Parmesan cheese
- 2 tablespoons fresh parsley, chopped
- 1 teaspoon dried thyme
- 1 teaspoon dried rosemary
- 1/2 teaspoon garlic powder
- 2 tablespoons olive oil
- Salt and pepper to taste

📋 **Instructions:**

1. Preheat the oven to 375°F (190°C).
2. In a bowl, combine breadcrumbs, Parmesan cheese, parsley, thyme, rosemary, garlic powder, salt, and pepper.
3. Brush the chicken breasts with olive oil.
4. Dredge each chicken breast in the breadcrumb mixture, pressing lightly to adhere.
5. Place the chicken on a baking sheet lined with parchment paper.
6. Bake for 25-30 minutes or until the chicken is cooked through and the coating is golden brown.
7. Serve immediately.

🍰 **Nutritional Information:** Calories: 350 | Protein: 30g | Carbs: 10g | Fat: 20g | Fiber: 2g

Quinoa-Stuffed Acorn Squash

⏱ **Prep Time:** 15 minutes | 🔍 **Cooking Time:** 45 minutes | 🍽 **Servings:** 4

🛒 **Ingredients:**

- 2 acorn squashes, halved and seeds removed
- 1 cup cooked quinoa
- 1/2 cup dried cranberries
- 1/2 cup chopped pecans
- 1/4 cup fresh parsley, chopped
- 1 tablespoon olive oil
- Salt and pepper to taste

📋 **Instructions:**

1. Preheat the oven to 400°F (200°C).
2. Brush the cut sides of the acorn squash with olive oil and season with salt and pepper.

3. Place the squash halves cut-side down on a baking sheet and roast for 30 minutes or until tender.
4. In a bowl, combine cooked quinoa, dried cranberries, chopped pecans, and fresh parsley.
5. Fill each squash half with the quinoa mixture.
6. Return to the oven and bake for an additional 10-15 minutes.
7. Serve warm.

Nutritional Information: Calories: 280 | Protein: 6g | Carbs: 45g | Fat: 12g | Fiber: 7g

Lemon Herb Grilled Salmon

Prep Time: 10 minutes | **Cooking Time:** 15 minutes | **Servings:** 4

Ingredients:

- 4 salmon fillets
- 1/4 cup olive oil
- 2 tablespoons lemon juice
- 2 garlic cloves, minced
- 1 tablespoon fresh dill, chopped
- 1 tablespoon fresh parsley, chopped
- Salt and pepper to taste

Instructions:

1. Preheat the grill to medium-high heat.
2. In a small bowl, whisk together olive oil, lemon juice, garlic, dill, parsley, salt, and pepper.
3. Brush the salmon fillets with the herb mixture.
4. Grill the salmon fillets for 6-7 minutes on each side, or until the fish flakes easily with a fork.
5. Serve immediately.

Nutritional Information: Calories: 350 | Protein: 30g | Carbs: 2g | Fat: 24g | Fiber: 0g

Cauliflower Rice and Turkey Stuffed Peppers

Prep Time: 15 minutes | **Cooking Time:** 30 minutes | **Servings:** 4

Ingredients:

- 4 bell peppers, tops cut off and seeds removed
- 1 pound ground turkey
- 2 cups cauliflower rice
- 1 onion, diced
- 2 garlic cloves, minced
- 1 can (15 oz) diced tomatoes
- 1 teaspoon dried oregano
- 1 teaspoon paprika
- Salt and pepper to taste
- 1 tablespoon olive oil

Instructions:

1. Preheat the oven to 375°F (190°C).
2. Heat olive oil in a large skillet over medium heat. Add onion and garlic, cooking until soft.
3. Add ground turkey and cook until browned.
4. Stir in cauliflower rice, diced tomatoes, oregano, paprika, salt, and pepper. Cook for 5 minutes.
5. Stuff each bell pepper with the turkey mixture.
6. Place stuffed peppers in a baking dish and cover with foil.
7. Bake for 25-30 minutes.
8. Serve warm.

Nutritional Information: Calories: 300 | Protein: 25g | Carbs: 20g | Fat: 15g | Fiber: 5g

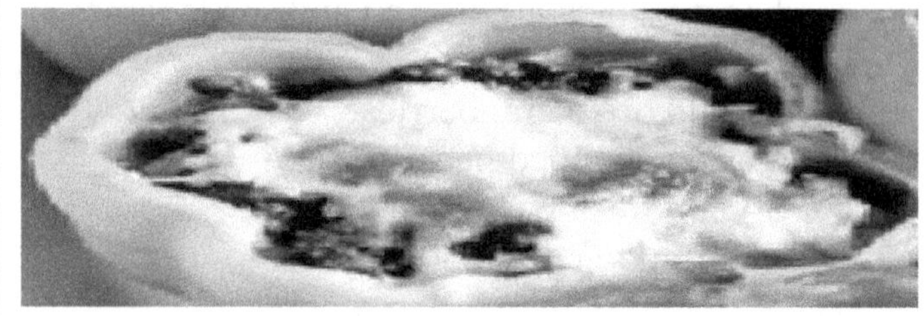

Zucchini Noodle Primavera

⏱ **Prep Time:** 10 minutes | 🔍 **Cooking Time:** 10 minutes | 🍽 **Servings:** 2

🛒 **Ingredients:**

- 2 large zucchinis, spiralized
- 1 cup cherry tomatoes, halved
- 1 cup sliced mushrooms
- 1/2 cup bell peppers, sliced
- 1/2 cup broccoli florets
- 2 garlic cloves, minced
- 2 tablespoons olive oil
- 1 teaspoon dried basil
- Salt and pepper to taste

📋 **Instructions:**

1. Heat olive oil in a large skillet over medium heat.
2. Add garlic and cook until fragrant.
3. Add cherry tomatoes, mushrooms, bell peppers, and broccoli. Cook for 5 minutes until vegetables are tender.
4. Add zucchini noodles and cook for another 2-3 minutes.
5. Season with dried basil, salt, and pepper.
6. Serve immediately.

🥗 **Nutritional Information:** Calories: 200 | Protein: 4g | Carbs: 20g | Fat: 12g | Fiber: 6g

Spaghetti Squash with Marinara Sauce

⏱ **Prep Time:** 10 minutes | 🔍 **Cooking Time:** 40 minutes | 🍽 **Servings:** 4

🛒 **Ingredients:**

- 1 large spaghetti squash
- 2 cups marinara sauce
- 1/4 cup grated Parmesan cheese
- 1 tablespoon olive oil
- Salt and pepper to taste

📋 **Instructions:**

1. Preheat the oven to 400°F (200°C).
2. Cut the spaghetti squash in half lengthwise and scoop out the seeds.
3. Brush the cut sides with olive oil and season with salt and pepper.
4. Place cut-side down on a baking sheet and roast for 30-40 minutes, or until tender.
5. Use a fork to scrape the flesh into spaghetti-like strands.
6. Heat marinara sauce in a saucepan over medium heat.
7. Serve spaghetti squash strands topped with marinara sauce and grated Parmesan cheese.

🥗 **Nutritional Information:** Calories: 180 | Protein: 6g | Carbs: 30g | Fat: 5g | Fiber: 6g

Baked Trout with Garlic and Dill

⏱ **Prep Time:** 10 minutes | 🔍 **Cooking Time:** 20 minutes | 🍽 **Servings:** 2

🛒 **Ingredients:**

- 2 trout fillets
- 2 tablespoons olive oil
- 1 tablespoon lemon juice
- 2 garlic cloves, minced
- 1 tablespoon fresh dill, chopped
- Salt and pepper to taste

📋 **Instructions:**

1. Preheat the oven to 375°F (190°C).
2. Place trout fillets on a baking sheet lined with parchment paper.
3. In a small bowl, mix olive oil, lemon juice, garlic, dill, salt, and pepper.
4. Brush the mixture over the trout fillets.

5. Bake for 15-20 minutes, or until the fish flakes easily with a fork.
6. Serve immediately.

 Calories: 300 | Protein: 28g | Carbs: 2g | Fat: 20g | Fiber: 0g

Quinoa and Vegetable Stuffed Tomatoes

Prep Time: 15 minutes | **Cooking Time:** 25 minutes | **Servings:** 4

Ingredients:

- 4 large tomatoes
- 1 cup cooked quinoa
- 1/2 cup diced zucchini
- 1/2 cup diced bell pepper
- 1/4 cup diced red onion
- 1 tablespoon fresh basil, chopped
- 1 tablespoon olive oil
- Salt and pepper to taste

Instructions:

1. Preheat the oven to 375°F (190°C).
2. Cut the tops off the tomatoes and scoop out the insides.
3. In a bowl, combine cooked quinoa, zucchini, bell pepper, red onion, basil, olive oil, salt, and pepper.
4. Stuff the tomatoes with the quinoa mixture.
5. Place the stuffed tomatoes in a baking dish and bake for 20-25 minutes.
6. Serve warm.

Nutritional Information: Calories: 180 | Protein: 5g | Carbs: 30g | Fat: 7g | Fiber: 6g

Herb-Roasted Chicken with Root Vegetables

Prep Time: 15 minutes | **Cooking Time:** 45 minutes | **Servings:** 4

Ingredients:

- 4 chicken thighs
- 2 carrots, peeled and chopped
- 2 parsnips, peeled and chopped
- 1 sweet potato, peeled and chopped
- 1 red onion, quartered
- 2 tablespoons olive oil
- 1 tablespoon fresh rosemary, chopped
- 1 tablespoon fresh thyme, chopped
- Salt and pepper to taste

Instructions:

1. Preheat the oven to 400°F (200°C).
2. In a large bowl, toss carrots, parsnips, sweet potato, and red onion with 1 tablespoon of olive oil, rosemary, thyme, salt, and pepper.
3. Spread the vegetables in a roasting pan.
4. Rub the chicken thighs with the remaining olive oil, salt, and pepper.
5. Place the chicken thighs on top of the vegetables.
6. Roast for 45 minutes, or until the chicken is cooked through and the vegetables are tender.
7. Serve immediately.

Nutritional Information: Calories: 400 | Protein: 28g | Carbs: 30g | Fat: 20g | Fiber: 6g

Lentil and Vegetable Stew

Prep Time: 15 minutes | **Cooking Time:** 40 minutes | **Servings:** 4

Ingredients:

- 1 cup dried lentils, rinsed
- 4 cups vegetable broth
- 1 onion, diced
- 2 carrots, diced

- 2 celery stalks, diced
- 3 garlic cloves, minced
- 1 can (14.5 oz) diced tomatoes
- 1 cup spinach, chopped
- 1 teaspoon dried thyme
- 1 teaspoon cumin
- 1 tablespoon olive oil
- Salt and pepper to taste

Instructions:

1. Heat olive oil in a large pot over medium heat.
2. Add onion, carrots, and celery, and cook until vegetables are tender, about 5 minutes.
3. Stir in garlic, thyme, and cumin, cooking for another minute.
4. Add lentils, vegetable broth, and diced tomatoes. Bring to a boil, then reduce heat and simmer for 25 minutes.
5. Stir in spinach and cook for an additional 5 minutes.
6. Season with salt and pepper to taste.
7. Serve hot.

Nutritional Information: Calories: 250 | Protein: 12g | Carbs: 40g | Fat: 6g | Fiber: 15g

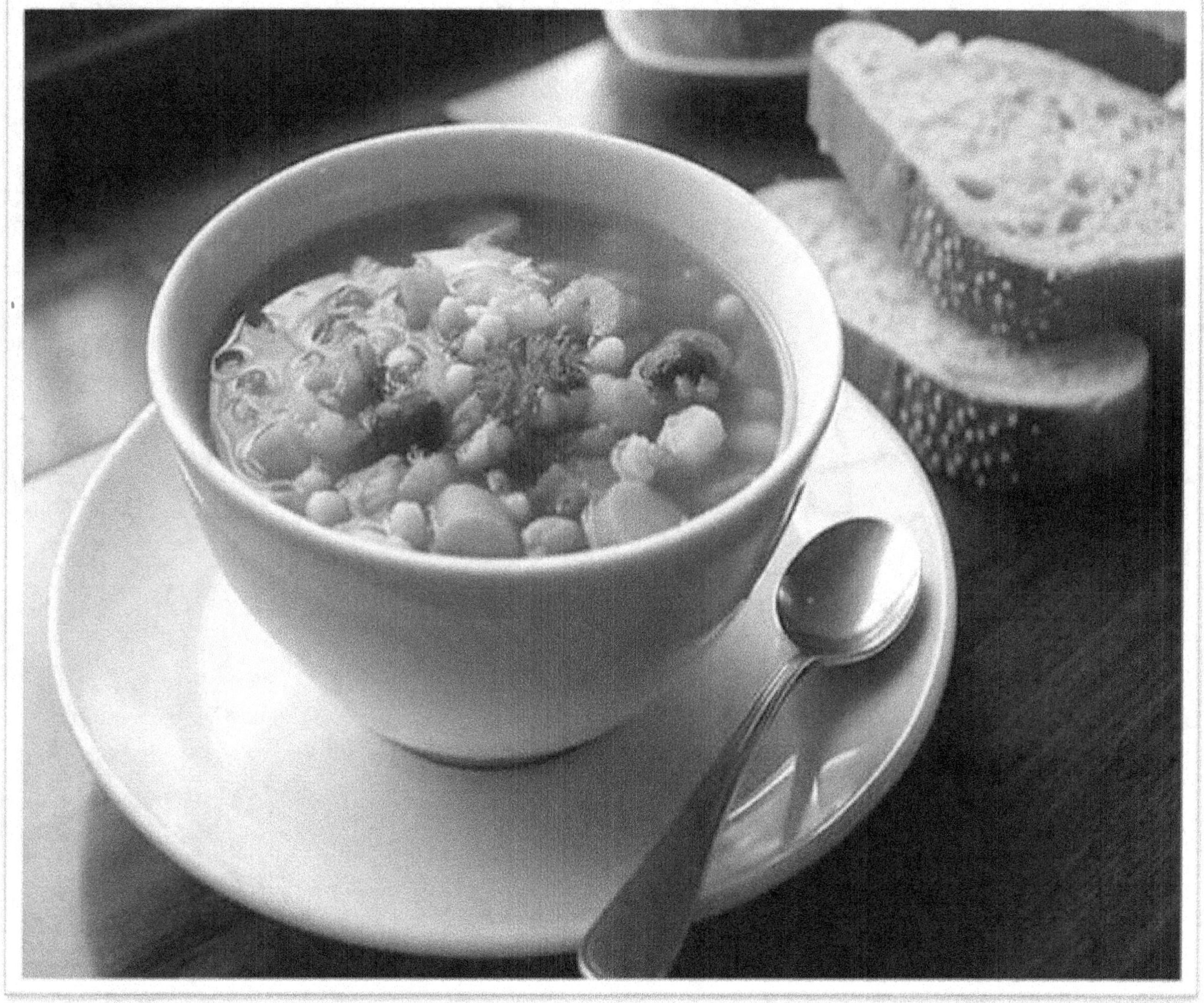

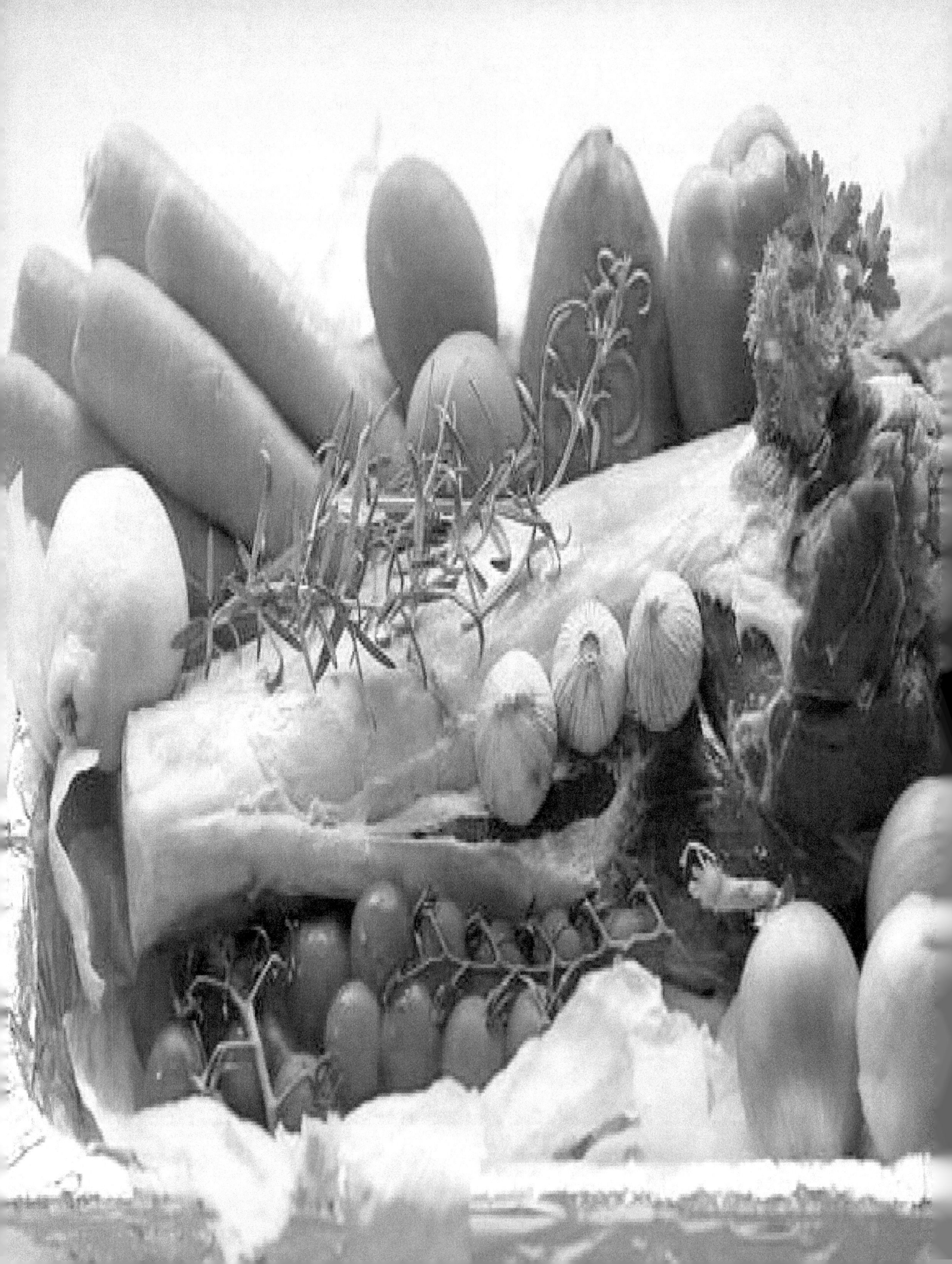

CONCLUSION

By following the recipes and general guidelines of this high-triglyceride cookbook, you can start eating healthier, feel better about yourself, and look and feel better to those around you. And at the very least, you will have lots of opportunities to make new friends at the health food store, and you may even find that eating low-fat, lower-calorie foods actually costs less than following your usual eating patterns. Are you convinced yet? Try some of the recipes on your loved ones, take note of how good you feel after making the change, then take advantage of your good fortune to show others that they'll live longer, healthier lives.

Tips for Maintaining a Low Triglyceride Diet

Important tips for maintaining a low triglyceride diet include:
1. Limit carbohydrates and increase protein.
2. Switch to whole grains.
3. Fill up with fresh fruits and vegetables.
4. Get more fiber to lower triglycerides.
5. Using healthy vegetable oils will lower triglycerides.
6. Eat at regular intervals.
7. Enjoy small, healthy meals.
8. Be mindful of portion sizes to keep triglycerides low.
9. Watch what you drink.
10. Avoid alcohol.
11. Consume alcohol sparingly.
12. Skip sugary drinks.
13. Especially, avoid drinking high-calorie drinks.
14. Choose Healthy Fats
15. Eat Omega-3 Rich Foods
16. Stay Hydrated
17. Plan Your Meals
18. Stay Active

Grocery Shopping Guide

1. **Produce Aisle:** Stock up on a variety of fresh fruits and vegetables.
2. **Grains:** Choose whole grains like quinoa, brown rice, and whole wheat products.
3. **Proteins:** Select lean proteins such as chicken, turkey, tofu, and legumes. Don't forget fatty fish for omega-3s.
4. **Dairy Alternatives:** Opt for unsweetened almond milk, coconut yogurt, and other low-fat dairy alternatives.
5. **Fats and Oils:** Pick up olive oil, avocado oil, and nuts for healthy fat options.
6. **Pantry Staples:** Have canned beans, tomatoes, and whole grain pasta on hand.
7. **Snacks:** Choose healthy snacks like hummus, fresh fruit, mixed nuts, and Greek yogurt.

Frequently Asked Questions

Q: What are triglycerides? **A:** Triglycerides are a type of fat found in your blood, used for energy between meals.

Q: How often should I check my triglyceride levels? **A:** It's recommended to check your triglyceride levels during your annual physical or as advised by your healthcare provider.

Q: Can I have alcohol on a low triglyceride diet? **A:** Alcohol can raise triglyceride levels, so it's best to limit your intake or avoid it altogether.

Q: Are there any specific foods to avoid? **A:** Avoid sugary foods, refined carbohydrates, and foods high in unhealthy fats.

Q: How can exercise help? **A:** Regular physical activity helps lower triglyceride levels and improves overall heart health.

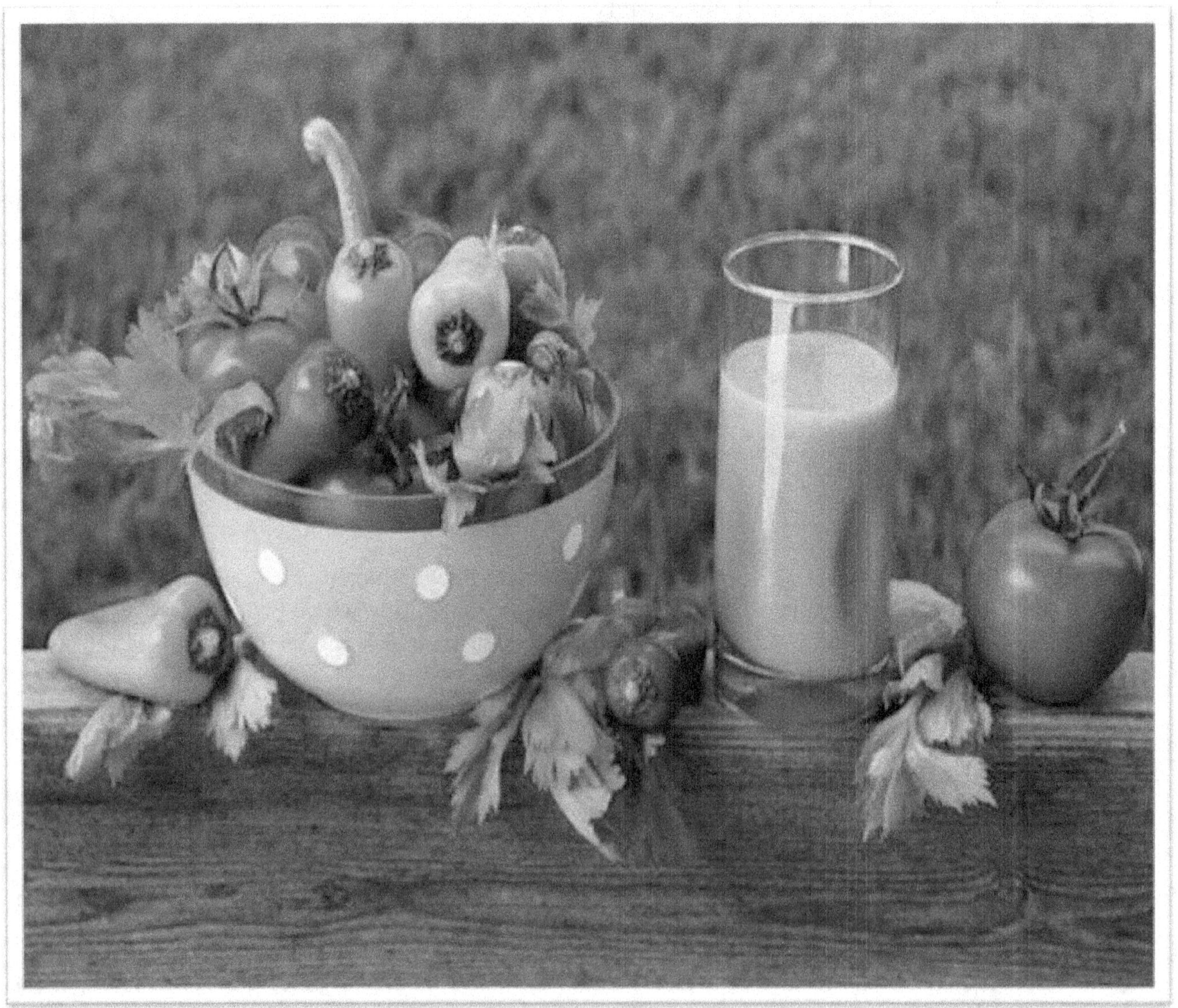

30-DAY MEAL PLAN

Day	Breakfast	Lunch	Dinner	Snack
1	Avocado and Spinach Smoothie	Grilled Chicken Salad with Olive Oil Dressing	Baked Cod with Lemon and Herbs	Apple Slices with Almond Butter
2	Greek Yogurt with Berries and Chia Seeds	Quinoa and Black Bean Salad	Chicken and Vegetable Skewers	Carrot and Hummus Cups
3	Oatmeal with Flaxseed and Almonds	Lentil Soup with Kale	Grilled Eggplant and Tomato Stack	Mixed Nuts and Seeds Trail Mix
4	Scrambled Egg Whites with Vegetables	Turkey and Avocado Wrap	Spinach and Mushroom Stuffed Chicken Breast	Cottage Cheese with Pineapple
5	Quinoa Breakfast Bowl	Spinach and Feta Stuffed Peppers	Brown Rice and Lentil Pilaf	Bell Pepper Strips with Guacamole
6	Whole Wheat Toast with Avocado Spread	Baked Salmon with Asparagus	Broiled Tilapia with Steamed Broccoli	Greek Yogurt with Cucumber and Dill
7	Berry and Nut Parfait	Chickpea and Veggie Stir-Fry	Quinoa-Stuffed Bell Peppers	Almonds and Dried Apricots
8	Veggie-Packed Frittata	Tuna Salad with Greek Yogurt Dressing	Roasted Turkey Breast with Brussels Sprouts	Celery Sticks with Peanut Butter
9	Green Detox Smoothie	Whole Grain Pita with Hummus and Veggies	Garlic Shrimp with Zucchini Noodles	Edamame with Sea Salt
10	Chia Seed Pudding with Fresh Fruit	Mediterranean Farro Salad	Herb-Rubbed Pork Tenderloin with Roasted Vegetables	Frozen Banana Bites
11	Avocado and Spinach Smoothie	Grilled Chicken Salad with Olive Oil Dressing	Baked Herb-Crusted Chicken	Apple Slices with Almond Butter
12	Greek Yogurt with Berries and Chia Seeds	Quinoa and Black Bean Salad	Quinoa-Stuffed Acorn Squash	Carrot and Hummus Cups
13	Oatmeal with Flaxseed and Almonds	Lentil Soup with Kale	Lemon Herb Grilled Salmon	Mixed Nuts and Seeds Trail Mix
14	Scrambled Egg Whites with Vegetables	Turkey and Avocado Wrap	Cauliflower Rice and Turkey Stuffed Peppers	Cottage Cheese with Pineapple

Day	Breakfast	Lunch	Dinner	Snack
15	Quinoa Breakfast Bowl	Spinach and Feta Stuffed Peppers	Zucchini Noodle Primavera	Bell Pepper Strips with Guacamole
16	Whole Wheat Toast with Avocado Spread	Baked Salmon with Asparagus	Spaghetti Squash with Marinara Sauce	Greek Yogurt with Cucumber and Dill
17	Berry and Nut Parfait	Chickpea and Veggie Stir-Fry	Baked Trout with Garlic and Dill	Almonds and Dried Apricots
18	Veggie-Packed Frittata	Tuna Salad with Greek Yogurt Dressing	Quinoa and Vegetable Stuffed Tomatoes	Celery Sticks with Peanut Butter
19	Green Detox Smoothie	Whole Grain Pita with Hummus and Veggies	Herb-Roasted Chicken with Root Vegetables	Edamame with Sea Salt
20	Chia Seed Pudding with Fresh Fruit	Mediterranean Farro Salad	Lentil and Vegetable Stew	Frozen Banana Bites
21	Avocado and Spinach Smoothie	Grilled Chicken Salad with Olive Oil Dressing	Baked Cod with Lemon and Herbs	Apple Slices with Almond Butter
22	Greek Yogurt with Berries and Chia Seeds	Quinoa and Black Bean Salad	Chicken and Vegetable Skewers	Carrot and Hummus Cups
23	Oatmeal with Flaxseed and Almonds	Lentil Soup with Kale	Grilled Eggplant and Tomato Stack	Mixed Nuts and Seeds Trail Mix
24	Scrambled Egg Whites with Vegetables	Turkey and Avocado Wrap	Spinach and Mushroom Stuffed Chicken Breast	Cottage Cheese with Pineapple
25	Quinoa Breakfast Bowl	Spinach and Feta Stuffed Peppers	Brown Rice and Lentil Pilaf	Bell Pepper Strips with Guacamole
26	Whole Wheat Toast with Avocado Spread	Baked Salmon with Asparagus	Broiled Tilapia with Steamed Broccoli	Greek Yogurt with Cucumber and Dill
27	Berry and Nut Parfait	Chickpea and Veggie Stir-Fry	Quinoa-Stuffed Bell Peppers	Almonds and Dried Apricots
28	Veggie-Packed Frittata	Tuna Salad with Greek Yogurt Dressing	Roasted Turkey Breast with Brussels Sprouts	Celery Sticks with Peanut Butter
29	Green Detox Smoothie	Whole Grain Pita with Hummus and Veggies	Garlic Shrimp with Zucchini Noodles	Edamame with Sea Salt
30	Chia Seed Pudding with Fresh Fruit	Mediterranean Farro Salad	Herb-Rubbed Pork Tenderloin with Roasted Vegetables	Frozen Banana Bites

<u>**WE VALUE YOUR FEEDBACK!**</u>

Thank you for choosing this book as your guide to managing high triglycerides through diet and lifestyle changes. Your journey towards better health is important to us, and we hope this book has provided you with valuable insights and practical tips.

If you found this book helpful or enjoyable, we would greatly appreciate it if you could take a moment to share your thoughts. A brief review on Amazon, along with a photo of the cover or a favorite section, would help us reach more people looking for guidance on this important topic.

Your feedback truly matters to us, and we read every review carefully. To leave a review, simply visit the book's page on Amazon, scroll down to the "Customer Reviews" section, and click on "Write a Customer Review."

Thank you for your support and for being a part of our community dedicated to health and wellness!

Warm regards,

<u>Cheryl C. Smith.</u>

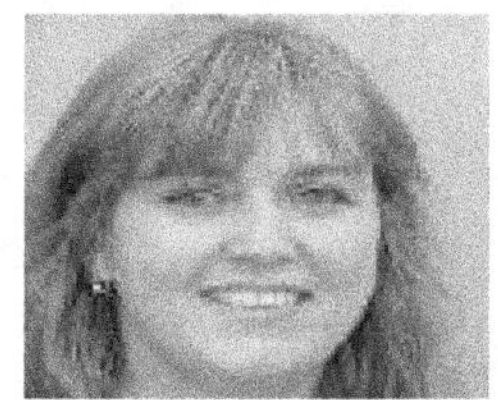 Dr. Cheryl C. Smith is a distinguished medical professional and nutrition expert who has dedicated her life to empowering individuals to live healthier and happier lives through the power of food. Cheryl's path began as a personal victory over her own health issues throughout her early years. She has a profound enthusiasm for nutrition and health. She overcame a variety of illnesses, from inherited susceptibilities to poor eating patterns, and came out stronger, equipped with the life-changing understanding of the therapeutic potential of nourishing foods.

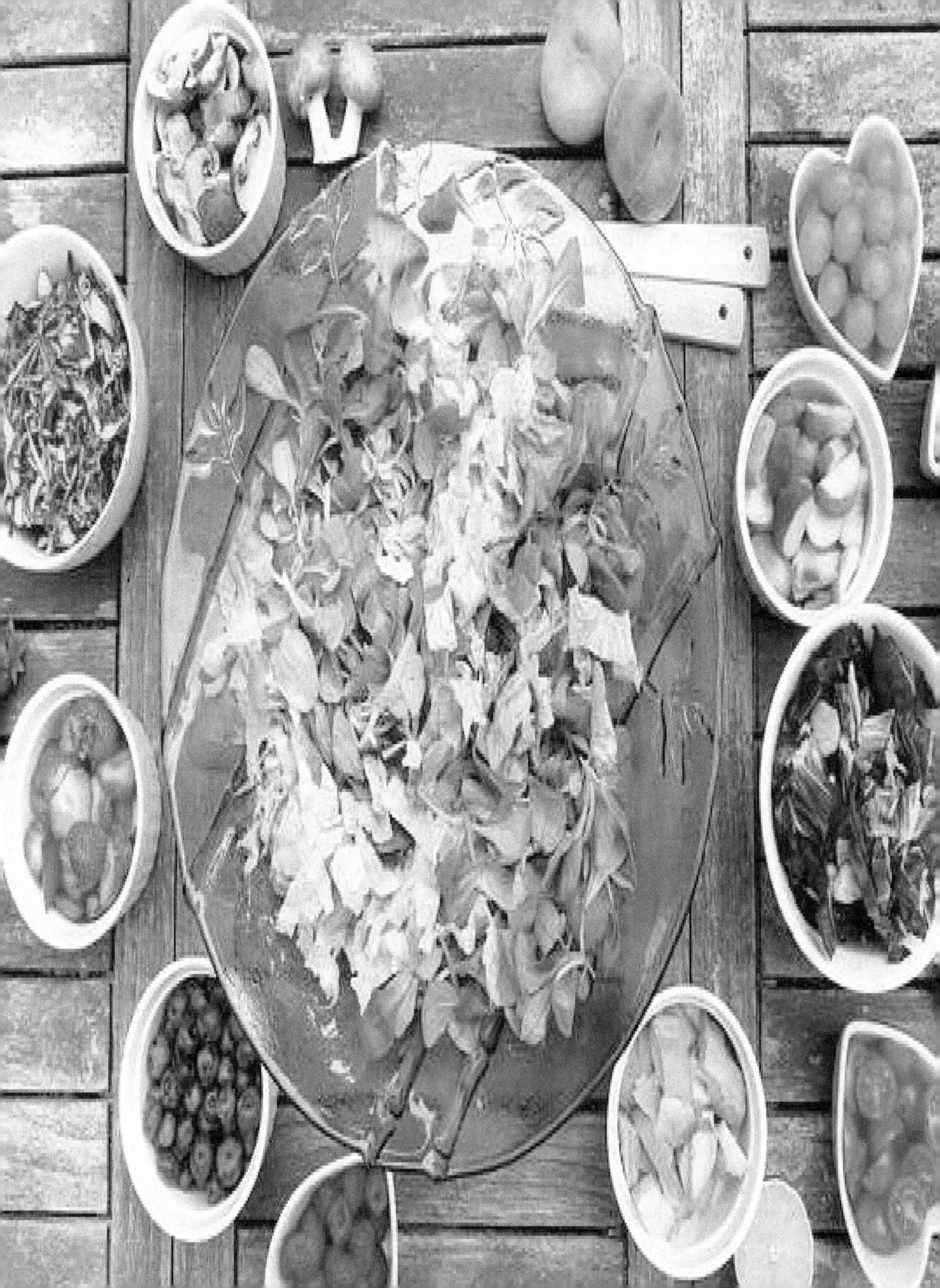

WEEKLY MEAL
planner

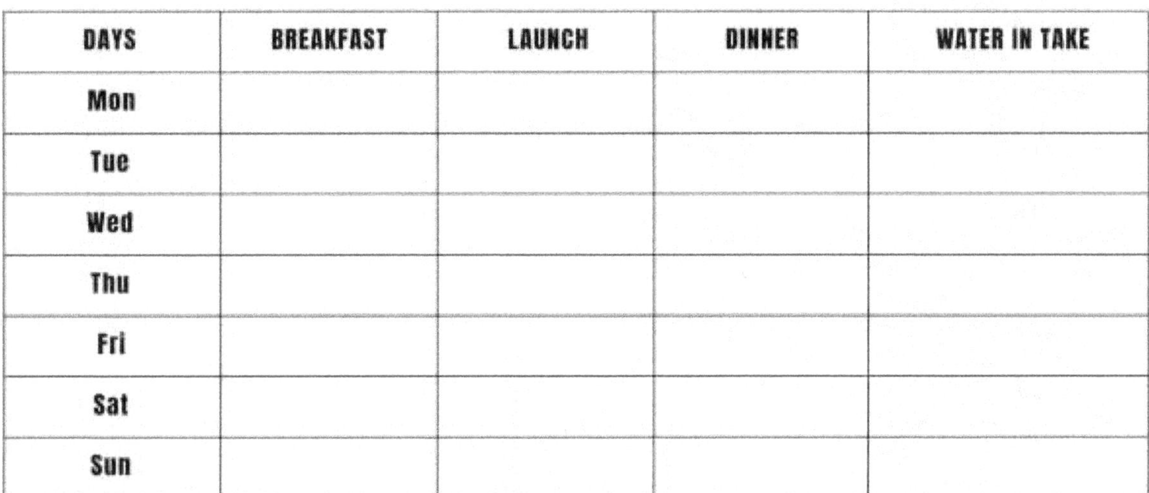

DAYS	BREAKFAST	LAUNCH	DINNER	WATER IN TAKE
Mon				
Tue				
Wed				
Thu				
Fri				
Sat				
Sun				

GROCERY LIST

TO DO:

NOTES

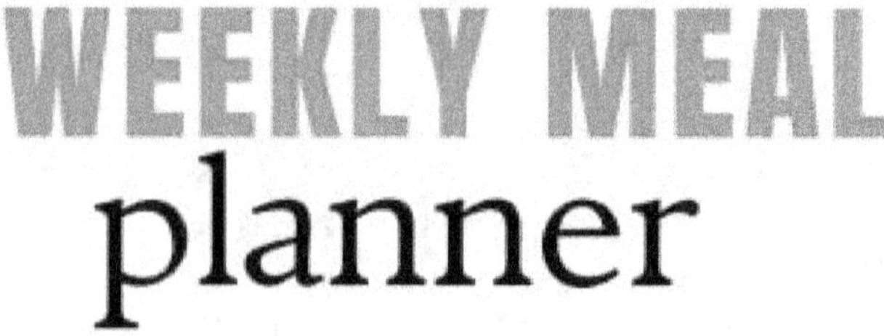

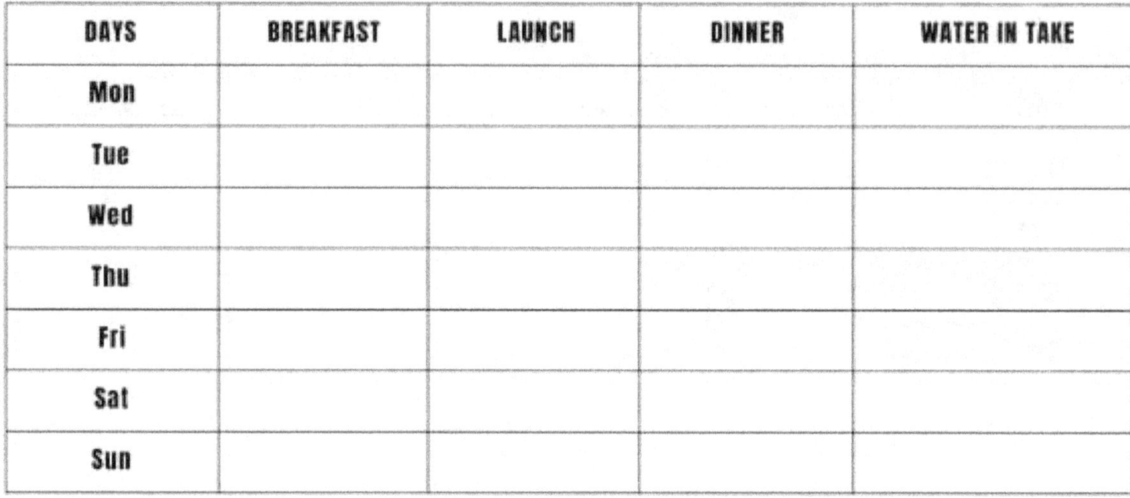

DAYS	BREAKFAST	LAUNCH	DINNER	WATER IN TAKE
Mon				
Tue				
Wed				
Thu				
Fri				
Sat				
Sun				

GROCERY LIST

TO DO:

NOTES

WEEKLY MEAL planner

DAYS	BREAKFAST	LAUNCH	DINNER	WATER IN TAKE
Mon				
Tue				
Wed				
Thu				
Fri				
Sat				
Sun				

GROCERY LIST

TO DO:

NOTES

WEEKLY MEAL
planner

DAYS	BREAKFAST	LAUNCH	DINNER	WATER IN TAKE
Mon				
Tue				
Wed				
Thu				
Fri				
Sat				
Sun				

GROCERY LIST

TO DO:

NOTES

NOTES

WEEKLY MEAL
planner

DAYS	BREAKFAST	LAUNCH	DINNER	WATER IN TAKE
Mon				
Tue				
Wed				
Thu				
Fri				
Sat				
Sun				

GROCERY LIST

TO DO:

NOTES

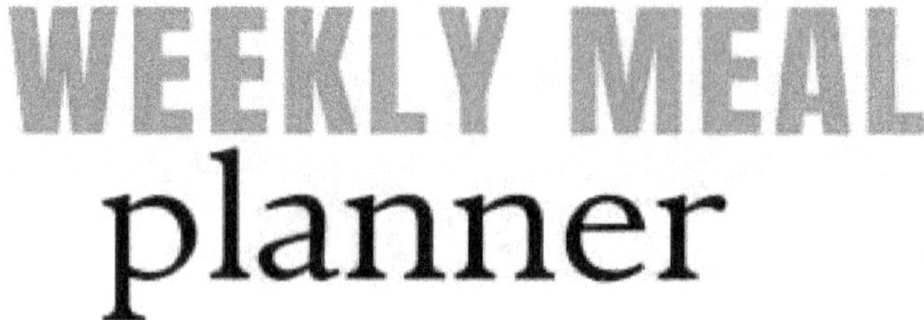

WEEKLY MEAL planner

DAYS	BREAKFAST	LAUNCH	DINNER	WATER IN TAKE
Mon				
Tue				
Wed				
Thu				
Fri				
Sat				
Sun				

GROCERY LIST

TO DO:

NOTES

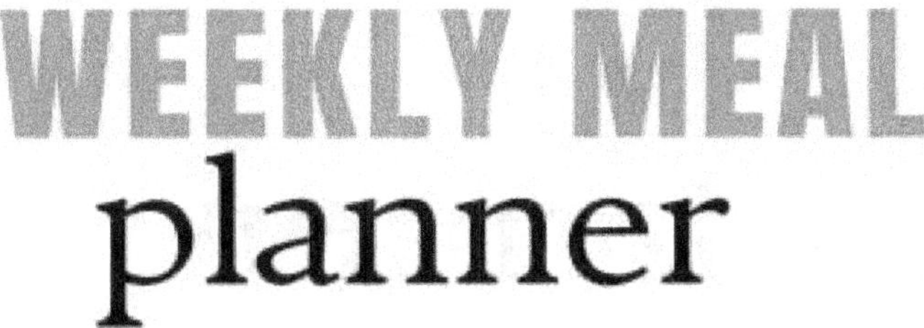

DAYS	BREAKFAST	LAUNCH	DINNER	WATER IN TAKE
Mon				
Tue				
Wed				
Thu				
Fri				
Sat				
Sun				

GROCERY LIST

TO DO:

NOTES

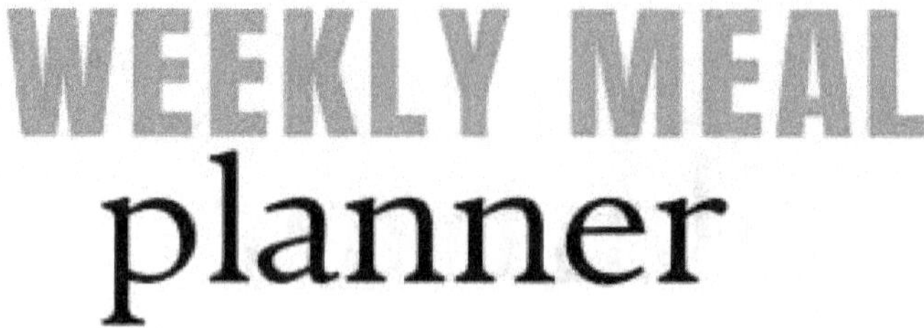

DAYS	BREAKFAST	LAUNCH	DINNER	WATER IN TAKE
Mon				
Tue				
Wed				
Thu				
Fri				
Sat				
Sun				

GROCERY LIST

TO DO:

NOTES

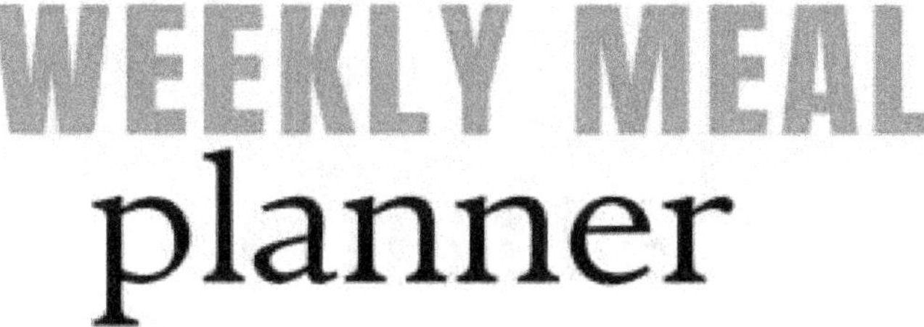

DAYS	BREAKFAST	LAUNCH	DINNER	WATER IN TAKE
Mon				
Tue				
Wed				
Thu				
Fri				
Sat				
Sun				

GROCERY LIST

TO DO:

NOTES

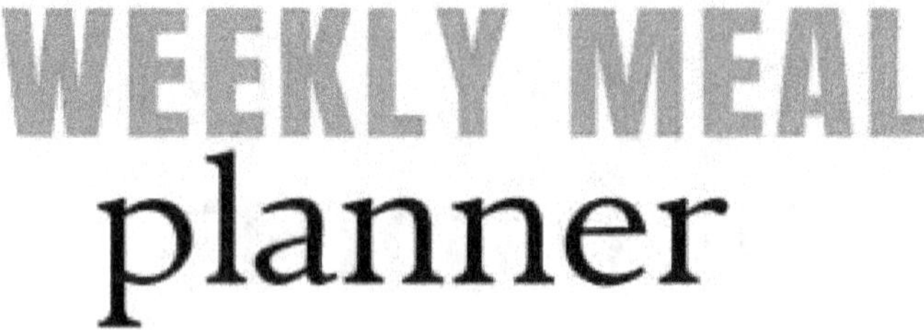

DAYS	BREAKFAST	LAUNCH	DINNER	WATER IN TAKE
Mon				
Tue				
Wed				
Thu				
Fri				
Sat				
Sun				

GROCERY LIST

TO DO:

NOTES

WEEKLY MEAL
planner

DAYS	BREAKFAST	LAUNCH	DINNER	WATER IN TAKE
Mon				
Tue				
Wed				
Thu				
Fri				
Sat				
Sun				

GROCERY LIST

TO DO:

NOTES

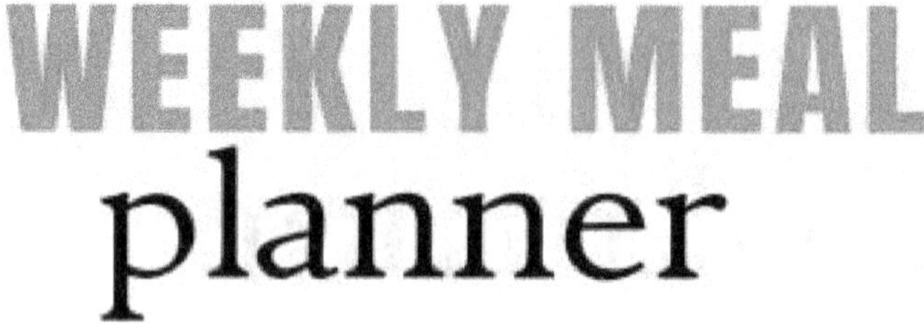

DAYS	BREAKFAST	LAUNCH	DINNER	WATER IN TAKE
Mon				
Tue				
Wed				
Thu				
Fri				
Sat				
Sun				

GROCERY LIST

TO DO:

NOTES

WEEKLY MEAL
planner

DAYS	BREAKFAST	LAUNCH	DINNER	WATER IN TAKE
Mon				
Tue				
Wed				
Thu				
Fri				
Sat				
Sun				

GROCERY LIST

TO DO:

NOTES

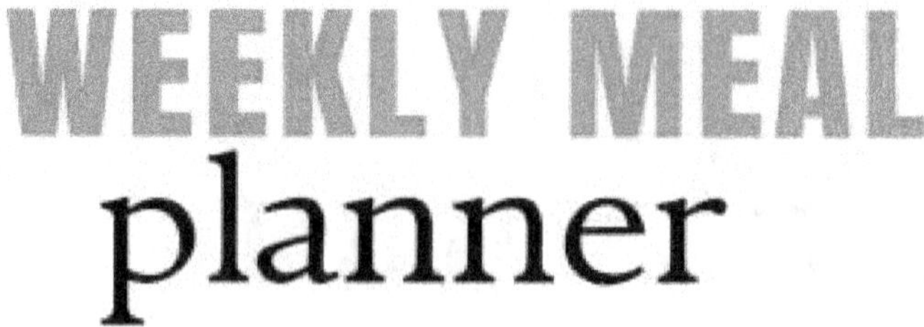

DAYS	BREAKFAST	LAUNCH	DINNER	WATER IN TAKE
Mon				
Tue				
Wed				
Thu				
Fri				
Sat				
Sun				

GROCERY LIST

TO DO:

NOTES

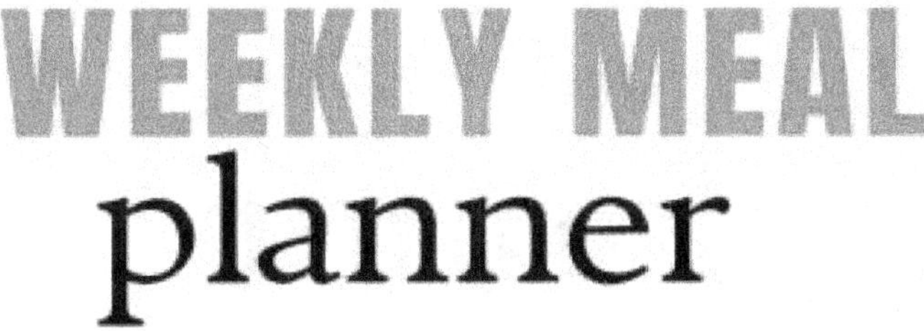

DAYS	BREAKFAST	LAUNCH	DINNER	WATER IN TAKE
Mon				
Tue				
Wed				
Thu				
Fri				
Sat				
Sun				

GROCERY LIST

TO DO:

NOTES

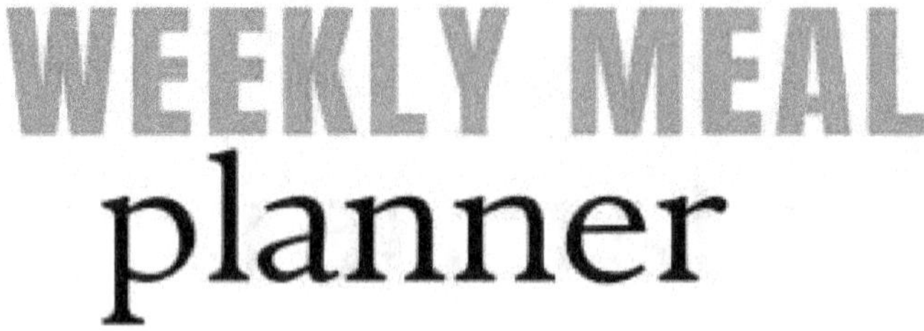

DAYS	BREAKFAST	LAUNCH	DINNER	WATER IN TAKE
Mon				
Tue				
Wed				
Thu				
Fri				
Sat				
Sun				

GROCERY LIST

TO DO:

NOTES

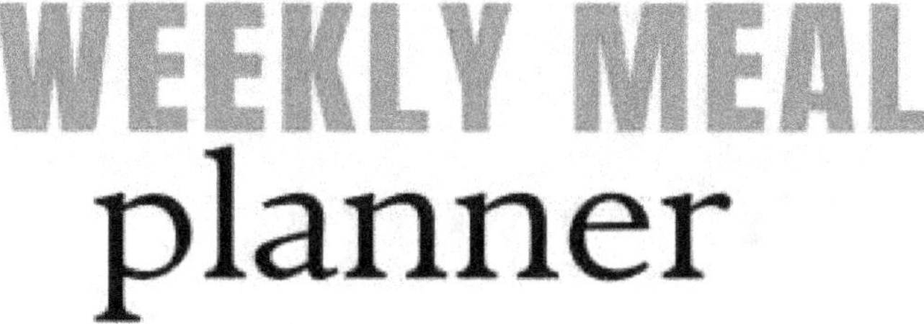

DAYS	BREAKFAST	LAUNCH	DINNER	WATER IN TAKE
Mon				
Tue				
Wed				
Thu				
Fri				
Sat				
Sun				

GROCERY LIST

TO DO:

NOTES

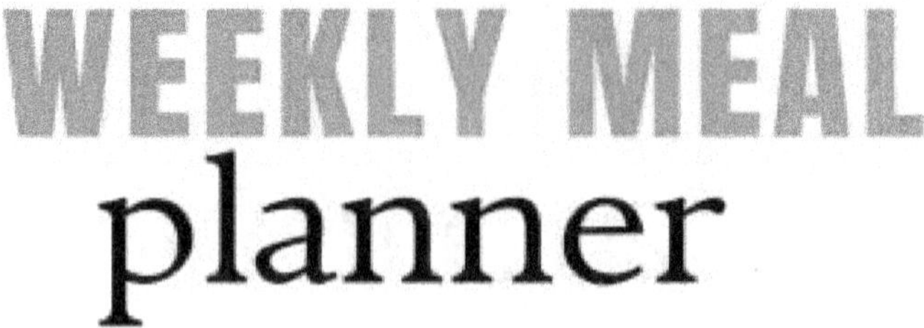

DAYS	BREAKFAST	LAUNCH	DINNER	WATER IN TAKE
Mon				
Tue				
Wed				
Thu				
Fri				
Sat				
Sun				

GROCERY LIST

TO DO:

NOTES